Vitalogical Hygiene

Dr. Johnny Lovewisdom

CONTENTS

Paradisian Publications
San Francisco California USA

Printed in the United States of America

CURRICULUM VITAE IN HEALING OF DR. JOHNNY LOVEWISDOM

Altho when he became a vegetarian, his first intention was to study at the University of Washington to become a medical doctor to teach others of the new better way of life, it became pointless if he remained at home with his family because of inheritance, if he was obliged to kill men in war for his country, so his first step was to forsake all of this. When he read the Bible after going to live as a hermit on Lake Quilotoa, he found that, the only one who heals was the Self, as already Dr. Clements had taught him earlier, Jesus told us, "Physician heal thyself", since what we wrote in the Book of Life by how we live was our only credentials. Yet with Dr. Clements' "How to Live" and later studies in other healing schools he earned worldly credentials for enrollment in studies, thesis examination or honorary degrees as follows, to wit:

DOCTOR OF METAPHYSICS: 1949, Brotherhood of the White Temple College Delaware, U.S.A., with Practitioner's Certificate in Spiritual Healing PROFESSOR OF NATURAL HYGIENE AND MEDICINE: 1960 Faculte Libre de France, Paris, and DOCTOR OF PSYCHOSOMATIC MEDICINE: 1962 by same. DOCTOR OF BOTANIC MEDICINE: 1962 and PROFESSOR OF THE VITALOGICAL SCIENCES: 1978 Honoris Causa, Brantridge Forest School, Sussex, England DOCTOR OF MEDICINE: 1970 National Ecclesiastical University, Sheffield DOCTOR OF NATUROPATHIC MEDICINE: 1970 and FELLOW PROFESSOR OF THE UNIVERSITY: University of the Science of Man, Hayward Heath, England DOCTOR OF NATURAL HYGIENE and DOCTOR OF PHILOSOPHY: 1966, Centro Estudios y Orientacion Professional, Seville, Spain. PROFESSOR OF NATURAL HYGIENE AND MEDICINE, PROFESSOR OF HEALTH and PROFESSOR OF THE SCIENCE OF MAN: 1966 Instut Philosophique, Scientific que et Technique de Culture Humaine, Bordeaux, France. PRIX. HIPPOCRATE for Service in Natural Hygiene and Medicine in 1968 DOCTOR OF SCIENCE: 1968, International Academy of Leadership, Philip. DOCTOR OF BIOLOGY, DOCTOR OF ANALYTICAL PSYCHOBIOLOGY, DOCTOR OF CLINICAL PSYCHOANALYSIS and PROFESSOR and DOCTOR OF DIETOLOGY: 1969, 1970, 1973 and 1976, Universidad Argentina de Psycobiologia Aplicada DOCTOR OF ORTHOPATHY and DOCTOR OF MYSTICAL ANTHROPOLOGY: 1973, Faculte Libre de Culture Humaine Integral, Bordeaux, France. FOUNDER-DOCTOR OF THE VITALOGICAL SCIENCES: 1972 National Ecclesiastical University, Sheffield, England The latter, National Ecclesiastical University, founded in 1916 graduated Medical Doctors, Dentists, Theologians, etc. who were authorized to practice in Great Britain and are true Apostolic Successors of the Old Holy Catholic Church, the Papacy in the Vatican State having been rejected by the greater part of Christians and their Churches. Founder of the INTERNATIONAL UNIVERSITY OF NATURAL LIVING in 1962, and on Sept. 18th 1975 as Founder-President of "The Pristine Order of Paradisian Perfection" it was incorporated in the Official Registry with Ecuadorian Government for the teaching of the Vitalogical Science.

INTRODUCTION

To understand any subject one must know precisely what is being discussed, that is, he must have the correct definitions to the words used. One of the first errors I was taught was in the study of hygiene and health in classes in U.S. schools. When I became a vegetarian due to my inner conscience and failing health, our text on Hygiene stated that one must not follow dangerous fads such as Fletcherism, Vegetarianism, etc. With the help of Webster's large dictionary, I learned that I had become a Vegetarian, and then going to various encyclopedias I was among the cult of the greatest thinkers of mankind, renown world champions in sports and holy men, yet these were called of a "dangerous fad". At least, the Hygiene books taught abstention, from tea, coffee, tobacco, alcoholic beverages and other health factors such as fresh air, bathing, sunlight and exercise and healthful habits, usually ignored by the students who sought to conform to the wayward social influence of their society.

Hygiene is derived from Hygea, the goddess of health of the Greeks, along with Asclepias whose cult was later assimilated by him. Thus Webster defines Hygiene (Hygienos Greek: healthful) as the "Science of the preservation of health; sanitary science; a system of the principles or rules designed for the promotion of health." In contrast, Medicine is defined as "Any preparation used in treating disease; the science and art dealing with prevention, cure or alleviation of disease." In other words Hygiene deals with health and healing, while Medicine treats only disease, in opposite and opposing perspectives. However, within the 100 years after the coining of the word Hygiene, by Hygienists, the Medical or Allopathic Doctors had surreptitiously appropriated hygiene for their own use ignoring the exact original meaning, so that vegetarian diet, fresh air, water, sunshine and many other factors needed for health were taught as dangerous causes of people's ailments. Thus, Hygienists like Dr. Herbert Shelton had to distinguish their teaching as "Natural Hygiene". With further infringement due to natural becoming ambiguous in its meanings often, Dr. Shelton coined the word "Orthobionomics", Bionomy dealing with the laws of life, Bionomics dealing with adaptations of organisms to their environment, so that "Orthobionomics" means "correct adaptations of life and environment". The latter addition of "Ortho" being necessary because ordinary biologists have no criterion to separate normal from abnormal, since Darwinian biology has defined evolution as adaptation, yet wrong-bionomic adaptations may be unhealthful leading to degeneration of the species. "Therapeutic" means to care for or treat in the art of healing, while later, the hygienists who sought to form their own school of drugless healing apart from the Doctors of Medicine, named their new adaptation Orthopathy.

Webster defines "Ortho" as meaning right, true or correct, while "Pathy" is defined as "Treatment of ailments of a specified mode, as in osteopathy".

Thus, in 1861 Dr. Russell Trall in his "Journal" wrote editorially: "The world moves. Since the establishment of the New York Hygio-Therapeutic School in 1853, whose professors are Hygienic Physicians, Hygiene and Health Education has become a prominent topic with many teachers and patrons of literary institutions. Amherst College in Massachusetts has led the way in establishing a chair for special instruction in gymnastics and Harvard is urging the appointment of a Professor of Hygiene". However, he complained that mere muscular exercises is predominating with a lack of emphasis in whole physiological necessities for health being ignored. So that the New York Hygio-Therapeutic College, the first and last college in the world to teach what is called Natural Hygiene began its existence. The degree given in this great school was Doctor of Medicine, and hundreds of men and women graduated from it during its period of existence and practiced thru-out America.

To understand why the above revolution in healing practices was required, we can best present them in Herbert Shelton's own word's in "Natural Hygiene, Man's Pristine Way of Life": "It was in an era of `hog, hominy and home-spun'. The North had just emerged from the age of white slavery; Negro slavery was in full flower in the South. In the West the process of murdering Indians and stealing their lands was still going on, a process that was to continue till it reached the blue waters of the Pacific, beyond which there were no more Indians to kill and no more lands to steal. Having thrown off the Old World Tyrannies, the New World was busily engaged in forging new tyrannies.

Grains, bread, pork and lard pies predominated the people's diet, vegetables and fruits were neglected, were contraband in fact. Nobody took baths, a strong body odor being regarded as a badge of merit. Fresh air was feared. Especially feared were cold air, damp air and drafts. Houses were unventilated and foul. No sunlight was permitted to enter them lest it fade the rugs, carpets and upholstering. Sanitation was neglected; tobacco was hewed, smoked and snuffed almost universally; alcohol was the favorite beverage and disease was common. The people suffered with typhus and typhoid fevers, malaria, cholera, yellow fever, summer complaint (diarrhea) dysentery, cholera, infantum, diphtheria, scrofula, meningitis, tuberculosis and pneumonia. The general death rate was high; the death rate among infants and children was appalling; mother's died in childbirth of childbed fever. It was a day of frequent and heroic dosage and equally frequent and heroic bleeding. In the South the summer season there was a cry of fever, fever, fever and calomel and quinine were administered lavishly, thus adding to the horror."

Medical historian Shryock states, "Unfortunately, the standards of medical education tended to fall during the first half of the nineteenth century. This was true in an absolute sense in the United States and at least relatively in Great Britain. In the former the rapid expansion of the population over a large area brought with it a mushroom growth of private medical colleges. Their owners interest in fees, or perhaps the limitations of their staffs led to these schools to shorten courses and otherwise to cheapen their degrees, and by 1850 it was easy for a man of no particular training to attend lectures for one winter and emerge a full fledged doctor".

In my high school classes, I enjoyed pointing out in classes the new knowledge I was acquiring studying literature of Dr. George R. Clements, who established the International School of Orthopathy, beside Dr. Benedict Lust, the founder of Naturopathy. "If all the drugs of the pharmacopeia were cast into the sea, it would be better for mankind, altho a bit hard on the fishes", I quoted from Dr. Oliver Wendell Holmes, contemporary American physician at the time Dr. Shelton speaks about above, 1809-1894. At the Philadelphia medical college professors of medicine taught they could give calomel to their patients and in the course of one tolerably successful season lay the foundation of the business of a lifetime, as they would ever after have as much as they could do to patch up the broken constitution they could make during that one season. Calomel in large and frequent doses was, at one time, the chief anchor of practice among allopaths. An old couplet has it: "Their souls were sent to heaven or hell by a doctor's dose of calomel".

So continuing the quoting of Dr. Shelton's superb description: "For at least a century strychnine was the best remedy the profession had for palsy, paralysis and paralytic affections. It was used to kill cats and dogs; it was deadly to hogs and cattle and, when given as a poison, slaughtered human beings. But when given as a medicine, it was a tonic, a nervine, a remedy for our palsied fellow man. Another favorite tonic of the period, one which was administered in all cases of fever and came to be regarded as a specific in malaria, was the protoplasmic poison, quinine. When McClellan's army encamped in the Chickahominy Swamps in 1862, his soldiers were fed on quinine, administered by physicians and surgeons as a preventive of malaria at the rate of $16,000 a day with corresponding rations of whiskey. When they became sick with malaria, their doses were increased. Never was a drug so unmercifully exposed as a failure, both as a preventative and as a cure; yet, the profession continued to use it and to swear by it.

There were fads in drugging then and now. Writing in the Journal May 1857, Solomon Fraese, M.D. said "A druggist said to me, There is not one bottle of cod liver oil sold now where there were 29 sold 4 years ago. Alas for the evanescent character of medical remedies! Alas for the reputation of medical men!".

Then Shelton tells of the medical treatment by fumigation of the lungs with opium, cubeds, deadly nightshade, iodine, calomel, corrosive sublimate, sugar of lead, belladonna, digitalis, hellebore, aconite, dogbane, tobacco, arsenic, antimony, niter, lobelia, cinnabar, etc. The miserable victims of tuberculosis, bronchitis, diseases of the throat, etc. died as direct consequences of such fumigations with poisons probably rather than the disease was the whole cause.

Writing on diseases of children, James Stewart, M.D., said, "The use of any medicine must, in general, be regarded as injurious, as the object of medicine is but to create a temporary disease for the removal of another; and only applicable when the disease demanding it is itself the greatest source of danger." It expresses the old fallacy contained in the choice of the lesser of two evils, except that in this one chooses both evils.

If fever was high and the pulse full, the patient was bled; if he was collapsed, with hand and skin cold, corrugated, pale and of a purple hue, he was bled. If a child was of strumous diathesis, delicate, frail and of feeble organization, he was bled. In low typhus fever and in collapsed cholera, bleeding was resorted to, to unload congestion in the large, deep-seated internal blood vessels. Blood was withdrawn quickly from the large artery to make the requisite impression on the body, as indicated by faintness, a train of morbid reactions could be broken up. If a physician was called to see a nervous, feeble, irritable, sick man, prostrated by overexcitement, enervating habits, depressing fears and loss of blood, he sought to help him by producing further loss of blood and more poisoning. It was even common to bleed in pregnancy to relieve symptoms. Bleeding was resorted to in case of apparent death from a fall and in other injuries. Bleeding was employed in wounds and head injuries that resulted in unconsciousness. Not only were pregnant mothers bled, but physicians also drew blood from blue babies. It was even the custody at one time to have oneself bled each spring and fall to preserve health.

Thus in January 1862 James C. Jackson, M.D., wrote: "Since I have grown to manhood, I can recollect the practice of bleeding being such that there was scarcely a morbid condition to induce relief from which some physician could not be found to advocate the practice of blood letting." He goes on to name a couple dozen common diseases to illustrate his point, adding "for every particular and morbid condition which could be found". This medical fad reminds your author as to nearly a century later, when he was at Modesto State Hospital his physician would ask the patient what his trouble was in the ward of some 30 patients, and then with report of examination of physical condition, prescribe penicillin beside the regular customary drug for the ailment.

Years later it was revealed that for certain conditions this could be fatal, or near so, and in my own case it destroyed the body's ability to produce the lacto-bacteria necessary for digestion in the intestines, making health delicate and putting to an end the 30 year abstention from dairy products to survive in optimum health. After paralysis produced by Parathion in a life working fruit orchards each fall, the treatment completed the paralysis until my body was a mere vegetable unable to move, with the prognosis of being two weeks from death, warning me in case I had to make a will, etc. This destroyed useful nerves to a point that only by training less efficient ones was limited use of the limbs regained when the penicillin shots were suspended and personally I was able to devise methods to seclude and discard the medication given.

Even this was frustrated, by an angry nurse who did not like my refusal to eat any beefsteak and meat on my special diet which I traded with ulcer patient who was getting my diet of lettuce, baked potato, etc. So the nurse went and got a syringe with insulin, probably intended for a diabetic case, shooting it in my arm cruelly claiming by this to give my needed proteins thru the arm. Going into insulin shock for days I kept rolling off the bed, henceforth losing the balance mechanism function of inner ear, and later giving hearing problems, making even relearning to walk of leg muscles and nerves impossible.

Soon there was another doctor who advocated the use of chloromyetin, when I was sent to the ulcer ward. Because of the side effects of the drugs given their were four flourishing ulcer wards, where the patients were rotting away with running sores. The chloromycetin specialists prescribed his new drug with such naturalness that one became convinced it was as beneficial as chlorophyll to hear him preach to disillusioned patients. I had already been disillusioned by the Parathion advertizing as an "organic phosphate", which confused one with the organic foods health movement. Any opposition a patient might bring on, was neatly challenged as pretending to know more than the doctors, and added to symptoms of paranoia. Worst of all, nothing was considered remedial other than the hundreds of poisons sold by the big drug companies. But let us return to basic errors of early 1800s.

During most of the last century, it was a standard medical practice to withhold water from the acutely ill and thousands of patients literally died of dehydration. The young suffering from fever would cry out for water and the physician would give them wine and even brandy. Due perhaps as much to the denial of water as to accursed alcoholic medication, the fever raged and continued and the patients died in great numbers. Harriet Austin describes a patient that was a stranger in a hotel: "He knew he was expected to die. He was tormented with thirst day and night, and not a drop of water could he obtain. To aggravate his suffering, he constantly heard a running stream of water at the corner of the house.

He watched his opportunity and crawled out of the bed and down the stairs, round the house till he found a large watering trough into which the water was falling. Into this he managed to get, and there he lay and drank all he wanted. The panic was terrible when he was discovered. He was placed in bed, clothes heaped on him and a messenger in haste to bring the doctor to see him die. Before he arrived, however, he was sleeping sweetly, and from that moment he recovered." But physicians continued to forbid water to their patients . In face of such overwhelming evidence, the profession refuses to accept anything that would threaten drugging.

This was a time when the sick were denied the benefits of fresh air. Physicians would give strict orders to keep the room closed and to keep air from the room. The weather may have been hot, the patient may have had a high fever, the room may have reeked with the odors of the patient; it was still necessary to keep the room closed. No breath of fresh air to be admitted. Patients were made to struggle in the confined air of their sick chamber.

Physicians were good at bleeding, leeching, cupping, blistering, purging, puking, poulticing and rubbing with ointment; but could not comprehend that a child cannot breath without air, that the parched tongue of the sick indicate the urgency of the need for water. Children and adults alike were killed by the thousands for want of the simplest elemental needs of life because physicians were prejudiced against what they called the "non-naturals". It was to protest against such practices that Oliver Wendell Holmes, himself a physician, but an avid reader of Hygienic literature wrote the following: "God gave his creatures light, air and water flowing from the skies; Man locks him to a stifling lair, and wonders why his brother dies." They classified drugs as "naturals". They classified as

11

"non-naturals" food, air, water, sunshine, rest, sleep, exercise, the emotions, bowel movements and writing in 1853, E. Mc Dowell of Utica, Michigan, said: "In 1840 under a popular Allopath I was fast sinking under fever. On a feathered bed, windows and doors closed on a hot summer day, pulse and breath nearly gone, I lay roasting. Friends stood around, looking at me to die. At this critical moment a woman called in to see me. She ordered both doors and windows thrown open, and with a pail of water and towels she began to wash me. As the cold water towel went over me, I could feel the fever roll off before it, and in less than five minutes I lay comfortable, pulse and breath regular, but weak, and soon got well". This is a typical example of the way in which windows and doors were kept closed and the sick were smothered in blankets, even tho it was a hot summer day and the patients temperature was very high.

Shelton concludes: Patients were dosed heroically, had their veins and arteries emptied of blood, were denied water to drink and fresh air to breathe and stuffed with slops. Is it any wonder that otherwise simple diseases were regarded as very malignant and the death rate was high? A real revolutionary situationary situation existed. The time was ripe for change. No mere reform would suffice. Should we marvel that the people lost confidence in their physicians and began (correctly) to suspect they were being killed by them?

So far we have relied on the foremost authority of our times on Natural Hygiene quoting "Natural Hygiene, Man's Pristine Way of Life". Now, for our humble supplement for the spiritually oriented minds we shall give our own perspective. Reading "Physical Culture" magazine in the 1930's and "Nature's Path", I noticed advertisements of Battle Creek Sanitarium" in Michigan claiming to be the Largest Sanitarium in the World, and Dr. John Harvey Kellogg was world renown as an advocate of basically Natural Hygienic methods including the vegetarian diet. His brother became famous as a manufacturer of Kellogg Corn Flakes and other cereals, today considered "junk" foods of a big supermarket business. This trend, originating in Hygienic origins, continues till today Loma Linda School of Medicine in California of Seventh Day Adventist Medical Evangelism, still graduating Medical Doctors, with some of the Hygienic therapy included, but due to the allopathic medical monopolism and restrictions are forced to teach pharmaceutic medicine. The vested interests have confiscated some of the basic hygienic practices which public knowledge has forced them to accept, yet remain controlled by the big pharmaceutical manufacturers, meat packing industry, refined cereals, sugar and other highly processed foods that have a long shelf life, because they are inert dead matter worthless if not harmful to life processes in humans.

Nor are the Bible Christians and Vegetarian Society people the inventors of Orthobionomics or Natural hygiene as they admit. True, Correct or Right Living is the Central or Fourth Principle of the Buddha's "Noble Eightfold Path, which all Buddhists accept. In that Noble Eightfold Path, he taught "the disciple must not accept raw grains nor flesh foods. Women and girls he does not accept. He owns no male or female slaves. He owns no goats, sheep, fowls, pigs, cows, elephants or houses." (The Word of Buddha) In the Surangama Sutra, he adds: "Pure and earnest monks, if they are sincere will never wear clothing made of silk, nor wear boots made of leather because it involves the taking of life. Neither will they indulge in eating milk or cheese because thereby they deprive young animals what rightly belongs to them... He condemns if they kill sentient beings and eat their flesh... I teach them not to cook their food even." If these facts are true, it is obvious that the early monks lived on mangoes, roseapples and other fruits, for which purpose such fruitful groves were donated to them. Then, the mention of monks begging foods such as rice and other cooked foods becomes superfluous. Either productive fruit groves or begging for devitalized cooked foods loses its purpose. What is most probable is that these original teachings against cooked food, have been interpolated to accommodate the later fat cooked food eating monks, especially with those of Macrobiotic modern trends.

In the Buddhist "Dhyana Paramita" we find: "Next in regard to eating. There are four ways of living. The first may followed by the great Masters of the great mountains, who live on herbs and seasonable fruits." However, as proof given by Western Christian observers, there is a statement by Hippolytus (225 A.D.) speaking about Buddhist missionaries: "There is among the Indians a heresy of those who philosophize among the Brahmins, who live a self-sufficient life, abstaining from eating living creatures and all cooked foods. They say God is Light", so in practice his true followers believed in Right Living, essentially as modern Hygienists do. Even the Buddhist shaving of monk's heads copied from missionaries visiting the Egyptians, shows an interpolation that turned monks into suspicious bands going around armed with sharp razors.

Altho modern scientists will concede that belief can cause many kinds of grievous psychopathologies, they remain skeptical as to what one may say or do as to religious faith giving one super-natural powers or even natural powers in the will to live indefinitely. The Christian gospel is full of references to Life Everlasting. There are also Buddhists with similar beliefs referred to in "The doctrinal culture and Tradition of the Siddhas" by Dr. V. V. Raman Sastri, "The Cultural Heritage of India" by Sri Ramakrishna Cent. Memorial, and "Obscure Religious Cults" by Dr. S. Das Gupta, which not only teach but illustrate how humans can be transubstantiated in body into immortal beings like the ones who now even still live in the forests of India who have surpassed a hundred thousand years. In fact, the Buddha and Nagarjuna are believed to have never died but as the Life of Buddha by Ashavagosha states, the Buddha could perform feats impossible to the mortal shell. Nagarjuna was believed to have lived 600 years, altho afterward he was believed to have achieved Perpetual Nirvana, in which Immortal Transubstantiation is understood as the emancipation from reincarnation, transmigration or metempsychosis. Metempsychosis is the mortal illness of belief and subjection to birth, suffering and death in mortal bodies indefinitely. As long as Karma is committed in evil actions those who die are only taking habitation in infant-bodies to accumulate more and more in the vicious cycle. So the true liberation of Para-Nirvana is from grosser forms of beings into perpetually renewed finer substance which also may be termed the ascension or resurrection from mortality. The Mahayana Buddhists thus do not claim they are seeking to obtain the unattainable freedom from the cycle of birth, suffering and death to selfishly gloat in emptiness, but as long as sentient beings suffer they shall remain vowed to liberate all. Such a body has all the powers mortals physically but at will can become invisible or be transmuted into whatever is needful for them.

As we have shown in our Aramaic translation of the New Testament "Buddhist Essene Gospel of Jesus", the Nazarite Master described by John, was believed by the Eastern Orthodox to have a body of super-natural or etheric substance, often disappearing in the midst of them, transfiguring, walking on water, etc. which is impossible to the mortal frame. That the Buddha or Jesus lived on cooked food, bread, rice, wine, etc. is contrary to living substance which requires life-energy radiations, showing the interpolations of monks in our Scriptures, since they lacked the full force living faith in their Teachers words. Far be it for them to live as public parasites, begging from door to door, but because the Buddha never accepted such haphazard donations of cooked devitalized food, the Sutras tell of their living in mango and other fruit groves donated to them for their sustenance and home wherever they preached. Likewise, Jesus began preaching at the Bethany banana plantation two miles from the great Jordan, where his disciples lived on carob, bananas and other sweet fruits, and later visiting Cana where they went for grape juice therapy, he fed the 5,000 on cake or fig-loaves of pressed figs, the living bread he preached about.

With this religious and philosophic rendering of recent times which made natural living impossible among civilized people, and our claims that Natural Hygiene was the teaching of the Buddha and Jesus, we wish to point out that Dr. Shelton's sterilizing of the teachings of the Bible Christians, Medical Evangelists, etc. based on religion, sought to make it purely scientific free of spiritual traditions. But now science is losing an aura of our faith and truth, since every year or decade it outmodes its past claims, ephemeral as the morning dew with no lasting foundation. Everlasting Life is based on the eternal law of nature whether Karma or in actions we sow today being recompensed tomorrow in future lives, life only begets life, or inert poisons taken into the body have no power to act, heal or cure disease altho the living body may act to expel them. Man's commercial research promotions sponsor the scientific education of our universities, making chemical fertilizers, pesticides, herbicides and food factory mechanization man's stand by, pharmaceutical drugs the basis of medicine, pollution generating factories, cities and transportation, economic barriers isolate nations and breed wars over business opportunities, and so on in endless havoc, due to the worship of so-called science. However, man is discovering that his Tree of the Science or Knowledge of Good and Evil should be known for its fruits, and return to the Tree of Life Everlasting.

NATURAL HYGIENE AND ORTHOPATHY: ORTHOBIONOMICS

Now, to survey the foundations that the Hygienic Medical School laid for Natural Hygiene, let us observe what Dr. Russell T. Trall said to obtain approval from the New York Senate to obtain funds to found the New York Hygio-Therapeutic College, the first and last college in the world to teach what is called Natural Hygiene. The degree given in this great school was Doctor of Medicine, and hundreds of men and women graduated from it during its period of existence and practiced thru-out America. Dr. Trall's exposition is as follows: "In a strict sense, Hygienic medication contemplates the employment, as remedial agents, for all purposes, except surgical, of materials and influences which have normal relations to the living system. These are: light, air, temperature, water, food clothing, exercise, rest, sleep, passional influences, etc.

"The philosophy of Hygienic medication is predicted on the primary premise, that those things which are constitutionally adapted to the preservation of health, are also the proper remedies for disease. It rejects from its materia medica all poisons,-all things whose presence in the vital domain is incompatible with the normal play of all functions, and which are destructive to the living tissue. It regards disease as disordered vital action, consequent on irregularity, excess, or defect, in the use of things normal, or as a result of the presence of abnormal things. And these propositions being admitted, it follows inevitably that the proper remedial plan is to regulate the use or application of things normal, and to rid the system of presence of things abnormal; in other words, to restore the normal condition.

"As disease is occasioned by the excess or defect of things intrinsically useful, or by the presence of things intrinsically injurious, the true healing art insists on regulating the one and removing the other,- and so relating the vital powers to all things that they can accomplish these objects for themselves, in the surest and safest manner possible. The fundamental problems which constitute the theory or science of Hygienic medication, and indeed, on which all medical science must be based, may be reduced to the Following:

1. THE RELATION BETWEEN LIVING AND DEAD MATTER

"Until the advent of the Hygienic School, it has always been held and taught (and is now held so and taught in all other schools), that, in the relation between dead and living matter, the dead acts on the living: that disease, causes of disease, poisons, medicines, foods and all external objects act, or make impressions on the living system. Diseases are regarded as positive entities. They are said to attack us; to have a course of their own; to run thru us, to affect or act upon certain organs; to be seated within us, to be self-limited; to travel from part to part; to become malignant; to assume a mild form; to simulate other diseases; to change their type; etc.; all of which language is consistent with the erroneous theory that disease is an entity, or substance existing outside of the organic domain. But it confounds the disease itself with its causes and its consequences.

The Hygienic School reverses this doctrine and thus solves the problem which has so puzzled and perplexed the medical philosophers of all ages. It teaches that, in the relations between dead and living matter, all action is on the side of the vital organism, and none whatever on the part of external objects. And in the solution of this problem it finds the rationale of all forms of disease, and all kinds of remedies, as well as the key to the interpretation of the problems of medical science, and all the rules and principles of the healing art.

2. THE ESSENTIAL NATURE OF DISEASE

The successful, or proper treatment of disease, implies a knowledge of its nature. The investigation of 3,000 years, have not enabled physicians to answer this question: "What is disease?" Its nature and essence are confessedly a mystery today. This is not the result of want of zeal or intelligence on the part of the medical profession. The subject has been pursued in the wrong direction. The solution of the problem has been sought where it does not exist. The observations of the medical men have been made from a false standpoint. Their experiences have been interpreted by erroneous rules. The data and the knowledge have been misapplied, and the world has always had a false theory of the nature of disease. But on the theory advanced by the Hygienic school the essence and nature of disease becomes self evident.

Disease is remedial action. It is a process of purification and reparation. It is not the enemy of the vital powers, but the struggle of the vital powers themselves in self-defense. It is not a thing to be suppressed, subdued, broken up, destroyed, conquered, cured or killed, but an action to be directed and regulated. To illustrate: when the body has been exposed to miasmas, infection, poisons, impurities of any kind, until the system, or some or more organs, have been dangerously obstructed, a special effort is made by the vital powers to cleanse the system,- to rid itself of their presence. This special effort, a remedial action,- is the disease. If this effort be directed to a particular organ or outlet, the disease is said to be local, as vomiting, diarrhea, cholera, consumption, diabetes, etc. but if it is directed more especially to the surface, or the emunctories generally, thus seeming to involve the whole system in the remedial process, the disease is said to be general, or fever; the particular form or kind of fever being dependent on the amount of impurity in the system, the vigor of the constitution, and the relative and comparative vigor of the various vital organs and structures.

Thus a strong vigorous person, with a slight degree of impurity of infection, would have inflammatory or entonic fever; a person of a more gross condition of blood and fouler secretions would have the remedial effort manifested in that form which we call typhus, or putrid fever; while the person of a more feeble condition and less impurity, would have the disease which is termed typhoid, entonic, slow or nervous fever; while the person who is contaminated with some specific poison or impurity which of necessity be thrown off thru the skin, would have some form of eruptive fever, as measles, smallpox, etc.

This exposition of the nature of fever suggests a plan of treatment which, for a quarter of a century, and various parts of the world and in the hands of physicians of all schools, and in thousands of cases, under the direction of nonprofessional persons, has been promptly and almost invariably successful. We, of the Hygienic School, do not regard the ordinary disease, (of which so many persons die every weeks, and which numbers among the recent victims the distinguished names of Cavour, Albert, Buckle, Hinckley, Douglas, Mitchell, Hoffman, Hawes, Summer,-all of whom we think, have unnecessarily died in their prime) such as fevers, pneumonia, measles, scarlatina, diphtheria, smallpox, dysentery, apoplexy, congestion, at all dangerous in themselves; and the mortality of them under Hygienic treatment, as I have ample data to show, is less than one in ten as compared with ordinary medicine, or drug treatment. Last week 49 persons are reported as having died in the City of New York, of inflammation of the lungs. That this mortality is chiefly due to the treatment, and not the disease, I most religiously believe. I have treated hundreds of cases hygienically, in persons of all ages, from eight days to eighty years, and have not yet lost the first patient.

If the process of purification is facilitated by proper regulation of the surrounding influence,- by furnishing the system with what of air, light, temperature, water, foods, rest, etc.; it can use under the circumstances, and by the careful avoidance of all injurious things, patients would rarely die of any form of fever, acute inflammation, or bowel complaint, known to the nosologies. Many of the Hygienic School have treated for years, all forms of fever incident to our country, without losing a patient, and, that, too, when deaths of the same disease were all around them, under ordinary treatment. But I do not propose to base the claims of our system to public confidence and patronage on experience; for experience is only convincing or valuable, according to the rule by which it is explained, all experience may be delusive. I rest its claims on scientific truthfulness.

3. THE MODUS OPERANDI OF MEDICINE

No subject has been more studied by medical men than that of the rationale of the action of medicines; yet to this day, medical books and schools, as well as teachers of today, confess that the whole subject is a profound mystery. The relations of remedies to diseases, or to the healthy organs and structures, are confessedly unknown, and are regarded by many as wholly outside the pale of human comprehension. We know that medicines do act, but how they act is entirely unknown.

The Hygienic philosophy reduces this mysterious problem to a simple truism, by reference to the primary premise,- the law of relation between organic and inorganic matter. Medicines do not act at all. Dead matter, I repeat, does not act on living matter. Drugs are dead inorganic, inert substance, and have no relation to living systems save that of inertia, the same as a stick or a stone. They are acted upon. The living thing is active, and the dead thing is passive. This is the law of all the universe, in relation to every thing which it contains. It applies to the drug in the human stomach, the poison in the blood, the elements around, as well as the medicine in an apothecary shop, the stone on the ground, the food in the field or the granary and the water of the spring.

The employment of drug medicines and the classifications of the material medics, are predicated on the assumption, that different drugs or medicines act on different organs or structures, in virtue of certain inherent, special, selective or elective affinities, which they, the drugs have and exercise for the set organs and structures.

The Hygienic School declares the exact contrary to be true. It teaches that living matter is active, and dead matter passive, in their relation to each other, always and under all circumstances. There is no affinity, and can be none between drugs and medicines, or poisons, and living structures. To illustrate: ipecac, antimony, lobelia, occasions vomiting; and salts, castor oil, galap, etc., purging. The popular system accounts for defects by referring them to the action of drug on the stomach, on the bowels, as its inherent affinity may elect or select any place or the other on which to make an impression. The Hygienic school explains the effects by referring them to the vital powers in expelling the drug, by the process of vomiting, the purging, as it can best get rid of them under the circumstances. Opium, alcohol, tobacco, etc.; are said to have a special affinity for the brain and the effect,- stimulation or intoxication,- is said to be due to their specific or selective affinity for an action on the brain and nervous system. The Hygienic School teaches that stimulation and intoxication are processes precisely similar to those of fever and inflammation, and the result is, vital expenditure, and vital waste, instead of accumulation or supply of vital power. The stimulation and intoxication, so far from being attributable to special action of alcohol, etc. on the brain, are commotions of the vital organs expelling them as poisons from the organic domain. In the struggle, this defensive war, which is nothing more or less than disease, or remedial action,- the brain is deprived of its usual supply of blood and nervous energy, the consequences of which is disorder, imbecility, or suspension of mental function.

These conflicting theories lead to diametrically opposite methods for treating disease, and as one of them must, of necessity, be wrong, the people have no interest as the great issues of life and death in knowing which is right.

4. THE THEORY OF VITALITY

The doctrine entertained and taught by all medical schools, except the Hygienic is that disease and the "vis medicatrix naturae" are antagonistic principles. The Hygienic School reverses this doctrine also. "The disease" is the vis medicatrix naturae. They are identical and the same. The life force-vitality and the disease, are not enemies at war with each other, each seeking the others destruction. But on the contrary both are self same vital powers in an effort to expel from the system injurious things and to repair the damages which their presence has occasioned. If this be the true theory of the "vis medicatrix naturae", that in practice aims to destroy the disease by means of potent drug medicines, can be nothing more or less than a war on the human constitution.

The difference between health and disease is simply this: health is normal action, while disease is abnormal action. In other words, health is the action of the vital powers in building up and replenishing the organic structure; or, in still plainer speech the conversion of the elements of food into the elements of the body tissue; and disease of the action of the same vital powers in defending the organism against injurious or abnormal agencies and conditions. Health and disease are, in the organic domain precisely what peace and war are among nations. One is a productive industry, and the other is destructive, but leads to a remedial action. Health is the vis conservatrix naturae, and disease is the vis medicatrix naturae. One is order, the other disorder.

5. THE LAW OF CURE

Here again, the Hygiene School finds itself in conflict with the dogma of all the other medical schools. Each of the drug medical schools profess to have the "true law of cure". But while they all differ in their technical expression of this law, the various phases are reducible to the same philosophical formula; which is thus stated by Professor Paine in his "Institutes of Medicine": "we cure one disease by producing another."

The Hygienic School teaches that there is no law of cure in the universe; that the only condition of cure, is obedience to physiological law. The popular medical system undertakes to cure disease by administering the causes of disease. The Hygienic system aims to restore sick persons to health by means which causes sickness in well persons. The Hygienic system restores sick persons to health by the means which preserve health in well persons.

The doctrine of the law of cure is founded on the primary dogma that nature has provided remedies for diseases in certain things which exist outside the living organisms; in other words, that the vital powers, when acting disorderly, are to be restored to order by the administration of poisons. I fear this doctrine has destroyed more lives than ever have been destroyed by war, famine and pestilence combined. The Hygienic School denies the doctrine that nature has provided remedies at all,- much less drugs and poisons. Nature has provided penalties to secure the observance of the laws; not remedies to do away the consequences of disobedience to them. Nature could not so stifle herself. (Hence) Providence could not be so inconsistent as to provide penalties for transgression, and then permit doctors to drug and dose away the penalties.

6. BEARING OF THESE DOCTRINES ON SOCIETY

As all art is the application of scientific principles to the production of specific results, there can be no successful healing art, unless it is founded on a true medical science. Physicians always will and always must practice according to their theories. They would be neither rational nor honest if they did not. And before they can have the correct rules for practice, they must have correct principles and science. The theory must be true, or the practice cannot be right, except by accident. And if all the fundamental premises of the so called medical science of the world are erroneous, as I have briefly shown, and as I would demonstrate if I had time and opportunity, no one need be told how uncertain, nor how dangerous, the practice must be.

+++

The doctrines of the Hygienic School; that all action is on the part of the living (vital) system; that disease is remedial effort; that medicines do not act but are acted upon; that disease and vis medicatrix naturae are identical; that nature has not provided remedies, and there is no "law of cure" in existence, are not only radical and revolutionary, but eminently reformatory. They dispense with all drug poisons in the treatment of disease, and find ample safe, and efficient remedies in normal agencies and conditions. They teach the world not to fear disease but to fear the cause of disease. They educate the people to do themselves no harm because they are sick, but to rest, fast, bathe, etc. until Nature, or the inherent remedial power, can remove the obstructions, and restore the normal condition.

+ + +

I said that these doctrines are eminently reformatory. Important as they may be in giving the world a better method of treating disease,- and establishing the true healing art on the basis of the laws of nature,- this is not the greatest benefit they are destined to confer on the human race. Far more important is their influence in preventing sickness. Those who become thoroughly indoctrinated with the principles of the Hygienic School, understand that, in order to preserve health, they must avoid the causes of disease, and this implies a life in conformity with organic law,- a strict obedience to every law which the Creator has implanted in the vital domain of that being which He has (fearfully and wonderfully) formed and fashioned in His own image, made to rank in the scale of being a "little lower than the angels" and endowed with eternal and godlike attributes. They must, in all things, "cease to do evil and learn to do well". They learn that a life which secures the greatest possible amount of bodily and mental vigor, which insures the longest period of earthly existence, which promotes the highest earthly happiness, and gives the utmost ability to do good in the world, is only to be realized in the use of all things of the universe, and in the abuse of none. And thus the teachings of the Hygienic School furnish the strongest incentives which can be addressed to human beings to live simply, healthful, naturally, and to be temperate in all things.

Abjuring the time-honored but most pernicious doctrine that life is a "force state",- a doctrine which practical recognition of has lead the way to all dissipation and debauchery in the world, and to a very large proportion of the vices and crimes which afflict society,- the teachers and practitioners of the Hygienic School are gradually, surely, and effectively exerting their influence in society, both by precept and example, which is in every sense beneficent and it conduces to the achievement of the world's first and greatest need,-HEALTH.

But aside from the consideration of better health, long life, greater useful-ness, and higher happiness, the Hygienic system is worthy of the people's patronage and encouragement on the ground of economy alone. Its adop-tion by the people of the United States would save, in direct expenses of doctors and apothecaries bills, not less than one hundred million dollars annually, and an annual and equal sum also in the indirect expense of the loss of time, business. Thousands of families and tens of thousands of intelligent individuals in this country and in Europe have adopted the Hygienic system partially or completely and have without exception found themselves less liable to sickness and more easily and safely re-stored when sick.

The Hygienic system has been applied, so far as practicable, to the treat-ment of disease, and to the conservation of the health, of thousands of of-ficers and soldiers of our armies and always with best results. Hundreds of valuable lives have been saved by it and thousands more with millions of dollars, might be if those of our wounded and invalid soldiers, who so preferred could have been permitted to have had physicians and nurses of the Hygienic School.

The Hygienic School is, perhaps, deserving of encouragement, as being the first, and thus far the only medical school in the world, which makes the laws of life and the conditions of health the leading feature of its teaching. While it teaches all of the recognized facts of anatomy, chem-istry, obstetrics, surgery, toxicology, and all other collateral branches of the healing art, like all other medical schools, yet, unlike all others it gives prominence to the subjects of vital development, physical culture, and personal habits, etc. which conduce to the preservation of health among the masses, and to the physiological regeneration of society.

And lastly the Hygienic School has peculiar claims on the munificence of the people of the Empire State as the pioneer medical school of the world in associating the sexes in the prosecution of medical studies, and plac-ing woman on a perfect equality with man in the duties, responsibilities and privileges of the medical profession. The policies which medical men have so long pursued of excluding her from educational faculties which the public, charity and legislative bounty have so liberally bestowed on her brother, is not only gross injustice to woman, but an outrage on humanity. Woman is, by nature and organization, by habit and domestic training, better fitted than man to take a leading part in the treatment of disease generally, aside from the mere performance of surgical opera-tions. Three-quarters if not seven-eighths of all the practice of the male medical profession is devoted to the treatment of diseases of women and children. And certainly, with equal educational advantages, women must be incomparable better adapted to manage the maladies and infirmities of children, and the diseases peculiar to her sex, than man can possibly be. In this line of practice there are no more successful physicians in this country nor in the world, than the women graduates of the Hygienic School. One, Florence Nightingale, has proven herself worth more than a regiment of male drug doctors in curing invalid and wounded soldiers of the masculine gender. How much greater must be her comparative success of the sick women and sick babies?

In conclusion, I will simply remark, that all persons, without exception, so far as I know or have heard, who have fully investigated the principles of the Hygienic medical system have come to the conclusion that they are wholly true." (unquote from Dr. Trall)

From the above presentation of the Hygienic School by Dr. Russell Trall one sees, to this day in the teachers of Natural Hygiene, have all been based on the unchanging laws of nature, and not on constantly uncertain change yearly in the "Merc Manual" on Materia Medica, or other pharmaceutical standbys of modern drug industries. What has changed among the Hygienists has been the use of terms to avoid confusion with drug medicine's methods, since their restrictions in application as even the Loma Linda medical school graduates experience, has made the drugless healing profession practitioners need to work under less dictatorial conditions among Chiropractors, Osteopaths, to exist.

ANTECEDENTS AND ANTECESSORS
TO THE HYGIENIC SCHOOL PRIOR TO DR. TRALL

To locate the original Hygienists and find the environment of the Pristine Order of Paradisian Perfection, in Mystical Anthropology we went back to the ancient Hyperboreans told about by the Father of History, Herodotus (5th century B.C.) whom he doubted to have existed in the description given by the Issedones. The Issedones were founders of civilizations living in the Gobi desert of the Tarim Basin having come north of the Altai or Celestial Mountains, home of the Finno-Ugric tribes which anthropologists have not been able to distinguish from other Nordic Scandinavians. These Hyperboreans were the first to say the earth was spherical, they worshipped the sun, their tropical climate allowed fruit production all year around. That this was possible in the land beyond the north wind, "Hyper-Boreas" has been proven in modern findings of mammoths and other animals frozen instantly with food still chewed in their mouths, showing a sudden change of the earth's axis so tropical climates have existed over all the earth. As Prof. Allan Walker of John Hopkins Univ. has shown with humanoid teeth unmarked in enamel, frugivorous man existed 12 million years ago long before the earth's glacial ages.

Hence as the writer of the Bible's Book of Genesis, as well as other racial traditions, thus all point to the Cradle of Mankind in north east Asia as anthropologists accept. So let us return to the relatively modern beginnings of science since Newton. Carl Linnaeus (1707-1778) was the Swedish botanist who invented the scientific naming and classification of the plant kingdom, declared, "Fruits and edible plants constitute the most appropriate food for man". Then, Baron Georges Cuvier (1769-1832), the French naturalist who was the founder of comparative anatomy and paleontology, stated "The entire structure of the human body, to the most insignificant detail, corresponds to being for plant eating". This theme we put across in this treatise that follows, since these men of science sought to prove their lives as vegetarians, not only involved the Paradisian Genesis of man's origin, but was spoken forth in the nature of man, his ethical reasoning in relation to the environment, kinds of food, structure beside religion and traditions.

Writing in 1852, Dr. R. Trall, said Dr. Isaac Jennings "Was widely known as the advocate of the 'orthopathic' plan for treating disease,- a plan whose details mainly consist in placing the patient under organic law, and there leaving him to the 'vis medicatrix naturae'. From the beginning of creation down to the year of Lord 1852, this method of medicating the vital machinery has eminently been successful and the personal experience of the author of the work before us demonstrated this also."

THERE ARE FIVE CLASSES OF SENTIENT BEINGS
DIETETICALLY SPEAKING AND ANATOMICALLY CLASSIFIED

We use the Buddhist terminology to avoid classifying thinking humans with animals, among feeling, sentient beings.

1.- OMNIVOROUS BEINGS: Those that eat almost any food indiscriminately whether animal or vegetable, such as carrion, flesh, grains, fruit and vegetables, completely mixing whatever they eat. The wild boar, domestic hog or swine are typical.

2. CARNIVOROUS BEINGS: Those that eat freshly killed flesh, fish or fowl, only adapting to other foods by lack or semi-domestication. Typical examples are tigers, lions and wolves.

3. GRANIVOROUS BEINGS: Those that eat grains, legumes seeds mainly with occasional use of vegetable or animal food. The dove, chickens and turkeys are typical examples.

4. HERBIVOROUS BEINGS: Those that eat grass, herbs and plants, sometimes fruit, even grains but refusing flesh, unless thru hunger and mixed with grains if it is introduced by trickery. The typical animals are the deer, horse, elephant and cow.

5. FRUGIVOROUS BEINGS: Those that live on juicy fruits and succulent vegetables or herbs. Typical of this anatomical class are the ape, gorilla, chimpanzee, orangutan and other anthropoids. The use of anthropoid should define resembling man, or man-like beings as having the true and original diet of humans.

Anatomically, man is inept for a DIET OF OMNIVOROUS Sentient Beings. Altho for many thousands of years civilized man has sought to adapt to eating all kinds of foods with impunity, yet it has caused great plagues of disease, short life-span and untellable suffering which he wishes not to acknowledge, unknown in his previous existence as a frugivorous being. Unlike carnivorous beings and Eskimos even without contact with civilization who prefer recently killed flesh, the American and European gourmet seek out well seasoned aged in months or even years carrion. Today his beef comes from flesh "alive" with moving cancer since the cattle are no longer living free on the range but are forced by hunger and confinement to exist on grains, produce filled with pesticides and herbicides, cardboard, sawdust, petroleum, sewage, etc. Likewise such omnivorous beings often resort to cannibalism since humans eat hogs, both living on the swill of all kinds of foods mixed indiscriminately.

(a) The saliva of the hog is acid, while the saliva of man is alkaline. (b) Man's intestinal tract is about 12 times the length of his body, whereas the intestinal canal of the hog is about 3 times the length of body. Since the hog's intestinal tract is shorter, it takes less time to remove the putrefying wastes, being less injurious, but even thus it dies before its allotted time. (c) the hog's incisor teeth are pointed and well developed, and adapted to kill and tear flesh of its prey, whereas man's incisor teeth are only fit to cut the tender skin of fruits and vegetables. (d) The stomach of the hog is simple and roundish, while the stomach of man is curved and has a duodenum. Thus man is not anatomically nor physiologically fit to imitate or live like the gross, voracious omnivorous hog.

Anatomically, man is not fit for the DIET OF CARNIVOROUS sentient beings. Man is not instinctively a killer, and only takes to killing for lack of food or superstition for survival among similar killers thinking it gives him added powers over his enemies. (a) The incisor teeth in the carnivore are very poorly developed, whereas the incisor teeth of man, those front teeth which he cuts tender fruits and vegetables, are very well developed. (b) The carnivores have pointed molar teeth with which he holds and tears his prey, whereas the molar teeth in the frugivore such as man, are blunt and adapted to crush and masticate fruit and vegetables. (c) The salivary glands of the carnivores are small and secrete acid saliva adapted to the digestion of meat protein, whereas the salivary glands of the frugivore are highly developed and the saliva is alkaline adapted to the digestion of the sugars and starch of fruits and vegetables. As a result of the different diets of the two classes of beings, the urine of the carnivore is acid in reaction and has an offensive smell whereas the urine of the frugivore is alkaline and has a pleasant odor. (d) The stomach is simple and roundish in the carnivora, whereas in man it is more complicated and has a secondary pouch or duodenum. (e) The intestinal canal of the carnivore is 3 times the length of the body from head to trunk, whereas the alimentary canal of the fugivore is 12 times the length of body. The short intestinal tract of the carnivore is necessary so the flesh food will not remain too long so as to cause auto-intoxication from the putrefaction of animal protein which produces cadaveric poisons. Meat putrefies quickly in a moist warm intestinal tract, so the length is 4 times shorter to allow rapid elimination. The length 12 times greater in the tract of the frugivore enables the extraction of finer nutritional elements that develop the evolved nervous system, brain and foster the spiritual development of higher beings characteristic of humans. (f) The colon of the carnivore is smooth and short, adapted for prompt evacuation of the putrefying residue of flesh food, whereas the colon of the frugivore is longer and convoluted, so that food not fully digested in the small intestines, undergo complete digestion and absorption before evacuation takes place.

Thus, one may imagine how dangerous and damaging partaking of flesh food is in an alimentary track that is many times too long for prompt elimination which putrefies and generates various alkaloids, ptomaines, leucomaines which poison the blood stream. Anatomically, man is not suited for a DIET OF GRANIVOROUS sentient beings. Without stone or metal milling machinery or cooking, salting, sugaring, and other process-ing, man does not find grains, legumes, seeds or the reproductive part of plants palatable and chewable, except large seeds and nuts, which con-sequently offer great resistance from being eaten. One finds this cracking black walnuts or husking and breaking open a coconut. Furthermore, al-monds and other nuts and seeds have poisonous skins even after shelling. It should make one wonder in the attempt to use them. Finally, a young man in full vigor of life will be astonished by involuntary or voluntary sexual desires and losses of fluids, so obviously man's first sins came by eating either nuts or bread made from grains. In old age or even youth a meal of nuts will give a belly ache due to the excess seminal protein. Nuts are unknown in the habitat of anthropoid primates being more suited for squirrels and rats. The sprouting of seeds (not merely soaking overnight) has developed a means of eating young vegetables from legumes, grains and other seeds, avoiding many of the adverse qualities.

(a) Grain-eating sentient beings have a gizzard, which is the posterior stomach of birds and fowls, which is provided with thick walls with pow-erful muscles and a horny lining for the grinding of food. The inner wall of the gizzard is so hard it triturates and grinds seeds and pulverizes sol-id masses of pebbles or glass in a short time. Even needles swallowed by turkeys, have been broken in pieces without apparent injury. The reason why fowls swallow such foolish things is to get something solid and hard with which to grind the hard seeds, since birds have no teeth. Nature has provided birds with a mill in a bird's gizzard to make seeds of all kinds suitable for food. (b) So man has tried to invent means to pulverize grains, legumes, nuts and other seeds, or cook them until they are bland and soft so as to be easily chewed and supposedly digestible. Man's gastric juice is highly acid and incapable of digesting starch, since this needs an alkaline medium for digestion. By the time the starch leaves the stomach and enters the duodenum to begin to digest with the alkaline pancreatic juice, the food is liable to suffer fermentation in the stomach and gener-ate carbonic acid gas which causes much distress. Since the alimentary canal of frugivorous beings, as well as the herbivorous, is too long for the proper digestion of starch, it undergoes fermentation; especially starchy seeds which are for the birds who have a gizzard. No food is verily man's natural food if it requires processing before it can be eaten. By grinding seed foods and softening them with intense heat man devitalizes it destroying food properties that make them suitable for birds. Thus cereals saturate the organism with calcareous deposits and become a prolific cause of hardening of all body tissues and premature old age. Birds need these substances to grow feathers, beak and horny leg covering as thus nature provides.

(c) Moreover, no other beings in nature are victims of the excessive stimulation and waste of seminal and menstrual fluids and the unnatural desire of sex for perverted pleasure in sexual abuse such as plague the lives of human beings. The habits of perversion such as masturbation, homosexualism, prostitution, promiscuity, and all unnatural abuses, retard and prevent higher physical, mental, psychic and spiritual development in modern civilized peoples. The useless production of excessive seminal fluids, and the shedding of menstrual blood are not found in beings living on their natural diet. As we have repeatedly shown in our courses on Vitarianism and Vitalogical Sciences, menstruation is basically an abortion, and seminal fluid cells are embryonic tumors, which engendered the cause of disease cells and organisms. Simple reasoning should tell man that seminal food substances such as nuts, grains, legumes, and other seeds give excesses of human seminal fluids and ova, and this causes overpopulation giving forth pollution and ecological problems. However, man is a slow learner, and prefers blindness to such facts. (d) The use of soybeans, peas, lentils, peanuts, mustard and other oleaginous and leguminous seeds are especially acknowledged in giving thyroid enlargement and consequent goiter. Just as cooking greens gives oxaluria draining the bodies calcium reserve, the use of seeds of any kind causes reproductive losses, and also other endocrine gland deficiencies such as goiter just mentioned, beside schizophrenia and other mental unbalances, accounting for wars, heartless tyranny, cruelty even under vegetarian rulers such as Alexander, Bolivar, Hitler etc. (e) The use of bread, nuts, and other seed foods lacking natural living water of a pure organic state, gives the need for earth water with inorganic lime, iron oxide, salt, etc. that stiffens the body with calciferous and other inorganic deposits giving hardening of body tissue and old age. (f) The cooking of grains, refining, removing germ of seeds, adding inorganic vitamins, minerals, etc. is further contaminated with white sugar, salt and irritating condiments to make them palatable.

Anatomically, man is not fit for the DIET OF HERBIVOROUS Beings. By mere accommodation thus ordinary grass can be rendered useful by man if by growing wheat grass or similar growing grass it is juiced free of pulp by artificial grinding to obtain the juice. Likewise, certain succulent herbs and vegetables are useful combined in salads, much like the herbivorous part of the frugivorous diet of anthropoid primates in their natural habitat.

(a) The salivary glands of man secrete an abundant flow of very alkaline saliva in reaction, and contain diastase to convert the carbohydrates of fruits into dextrine; whereas the salivary glands of herbivorous animals, such as the horse, cow, elephant, etc. secrete less alkaline saliva deficient or lacking in diastase. Grass being the natural food of the herbivore contains practically no starch, so it is not necessary for Nature to provide any starch splitting diastase in the saliva of such animals. Starch and sugar have to be converted into glucose and levulose before they can be assimilated, therefore Nature provides frugivorous beings with ferment diastase of ptyalin in their saliva. (b) The stomach of herbivorous animals is divided into three compartments and in the camel and other animals into four compartments; whereas the stomach of frugivorous beings is divided into only a large receptacle called the stomach proper, and the smaller compartment called the duodenum or second stomach. The various compartments of the stomach of herbivorous animals are adapted for the complicated and laborious digestion of grass, herbs and plants, all of which are rough, fibrous foods. The main stomach of the frugivore, as well as the smaller compartment, the duodenum are adapted both structurally and chemically for the digestion of the soft pulp of fresh juicy fruits and tender succulent vegetables or herbs and not for the digestion of hard fiber grass and straw and tree shoots.

(c) The length of the intestinal canal of the herbivore is ten times the length of their body, while the frugivore has an intestinal canal of 12 times the length of their body. Thus tough fibrous food is less suited for the frugivore. Man, seeking to avoid this cooks tough, fibrous food to make it soft, but this destroys the enzymes vitamins and organic minerals, adding work that wears out the deficient organism. The purpose of a longer intestinal tract is to extract all the needed food elements, but in an exclusive raw vegetable diet is constipated with the fiber after the juice is extracted. Thus various teachers like your author, advocated raw or live juice therapy to eliminate the fiber. However, the extremely alkalizing effect and replenishing of deficiencies, and sweeping out of deposits of accumulated waste products is good in the transition period, until the mixed succulent herb and fruit diet of the frugivorous becomes feasible. That one becomes light and thin on just vegetables need not mean he is undernourished since green plants are most nourishing in amino acids, minerals, vitamins, and enzymes, but rather one is not accumulating fat and thus thin and swift like a deer.

Anatomically, man is not fit for anything less than a DIET OF FRUGIV-OROUS Beings. For centuries since the first basic finding on the sciences, it was assumed that the frugivorous anthropoids lived on fruit and nuts, which is not true. The Encyclopedia Britannica under primates, subheading Diet, it describes 67% of the Chimpanzee diet as being juicy fruits, 62% of the Gibbons diet being fruits, 50% of the Orangutans diet being fruit and only 15% at the most consisting of fruits in the diet of the Gorilla. Their daily herb staples are bedstraw (Galius), wild celery, thistles, borage, nettles and bamboo shoots. If they find bananas they prefer the pith of the banana plant stem to the fruit. There are no nuts in their habitat, nor do they eat (as a regular diet or large proportion of their diet) eggs, insects, mice or other animal proteins, as some authorities on diet have supposed.

The erroneous view of nutritional scientists started perhaps with Linnaeus who wrote: "Man lives a natural life in the tropics, and supports himself with the fruit of the palm tree. He is only existing in other parts of the world and lives miserably on grains, tubers and meats." However the Nutritionist Dr. Sherman observed the experiments made by Dr. Jaffa with a group of California vegetarians which proved the average coefficient of their of fruit and nuts diet in digestibility to be as follows: for protein, 90% for fat 85%; and for carbohydrates 95%. Comments by Dr. Sherman were: "The fact that consistent vegetarians both adult and children, maintain a well nourished condition on diets of fruit and nuts which are of moderate total food value and low protein content is strong evidence the protein of nuts and fruits must be well digested and also efficiently utilized in metabolism. This in harmony with the belief that man is descended from ancestors whose chief food was fruit and nuts, and with the results of modern investigators of the chemical structure of nut proteins." The dieticians referred to are Mendel, Osborne, Cajori, Johns and Finke, as well as Darwin who theorized man descended from anthropoids. Yet, none of these suspected that complete protein or essential amino acids are supplied with green leafy vegetables, or the jungle greens anthropoids live upon in their natural habitat. The romantic Coconut Islands and Date Palm oases are still extremes to the true home.

(a) All sentient beings whose natural food grows on trees, are provided with limbs adapted to climbing trees and picking their food as well as searching for food in greens found foraging on the ground. (b) Of all animals, only the anthropoid apes assume the erect posture as man does. (c) Of all animals, only the ape's eyes look forward as man's eyes do. The eyes of all other animals look sideways. (d) Of all animals, only the apes and some species of monkeys have fingers in their hands similar to those of man. These fingers are adapted to grab, pick and pluck the fruit as well as greens avoiding spines and other obstacles. (e) In structure and function, the organs of the ape are analogous to those of man. There is a close analogy in every organ and tissue between the ape and man. The teeth, salivary glands, stomach, liver, pancreas, length of alimentary canal, in fact every organ in the body of man has its analogous counterpart in the body of the ape, thus, all these uncontrovertible facts prove that man's only natural food is juicy fruits and succulent herbs or greens.

For an anthropological perspective, as to whether before the glacial ice ages of earth, man was living as a fruitarian, Prof. Allan Walker of John Hopkins University claims he has found convincing proof that hominoid tooth enamel was unmarked which could only exist if the diet consisted of juicy fruits. He pointed out that the mentioned hominoids did not eat nuts, roots or the flesh of animals which wear and mark the enamel. Even worse are grains eaten parched and cooked foods which destroy the elements necessary for healthy teeth.

Now, as we recorded in "Mystical Anthropology" (Copyright 1979, International Univ. Press), man, the grain-eater has only miserably existed on earth about ten thousand years according to the dating of Anthropologist R.D. McCracken of UCLA. This we show must have started when the Tarim Basin and the Gobi Desert was the fertile Cradle of Civilization, and the "staff of life" or "daily bread" that man prayed for, began destroying the forest covering our green earth from there westward. It was a fearful thing to contemplate watching the new desert wasteland starting from the Gobi, then Mesopotamia, Arabia, North Africa, Europe, the Inca empire, the dust bowl of the United States, and soon if not curbed the Amazon Basin, swallowing up cultivatable food-producing trees, just for the sake of granivorous and beef-producing farmlands of an ephemeral duration compared to the earth's existence. Even worse, the bread, tasteless porridge and flesh food are the very cauldron of man's ailments.

Ann Wigmore and Viktoras Kulvinskas have illustrated how most of the ailments of modern life can be eliminated by turning grains back into grass and eliminating the cooking and refining of food, drinking wheatgrass juice and using legumes and other seeds to grow vegetables for salads, which really makes our "staff of life", baked bread, cooked foods and flesh foods being the "staff of sickness, old age and death". It seems unbelievable that for merely 10,000 years man has stuck to this passing fad in his at least 12 million years life on earth, or one one-hundredth (1%) of his frugivorous mainstay in earthlife. In the face of destroying the fertile earth to grow grains and animal flesh, and the multitudinous ailments starting his auto-intoxication, man persists in slaving his life away "in the sweat of his face" creating his problems of pollution of environment and basic overpopulation that such food engenders. Moreover, even if he wakes up to the need to give up flesh eating for the sake of economic, health and ethical reasons, he is still burdened with the long held belief that excessive proteins and starches are necessary, or that an all-raw or live food diet is impractical for beings raised on civilized customary concentrated foodstuffs, rather than fruits and vegetables of a high living water, enzyme, vitamin and mineral content.

In "The Recovery of Culture" by Henry Bailey Stevens, he charted the age of food bearing trees as a hundred million years, the age of the primate family as 60 million years, the age of anthropoids as 30 million years and the age of man as 1 million years. Prof. Allan Walker's date of 12 million years for man remedies the perspective slightly to the better. But the whole of modern science is topsy-turvy, inverted, due to Darwin's theory of evolution seeking to overthrow the Law of Disintegration of matter, Devolution in the case of man. The first man was the ideal integrated male with female, which disintegrated into male and female of our species, after eating seminal food-substance from the Tree of the Science of Good and Evil. Furthermore, "Adam named his wife, Eve, because she was the mother of all the Living." Because man ate the seed of trees, instead of the succulent herbs and juicy fruits of the Tree of Life, he disintegrated into males that toiled by the sweat of their face and females that sorrow was multiplied by conceptions and childbearing.

Obviously, humans can degenerate into animal-like creatures such as the gazelle-boy who could run 40 miles an hour along side a jeep using all fours and eat only herbs and tender roots, the ape-man living in trees like an ape, and so forth adapting to the peculiarities and anatomy of their companion animals if raised among them since infancy. However who has ever seen or heard of animals, without human selection and guidance evolve into humans. Clements, Goldwasser, and the followers of the School of Orthopathy, beside Herbert Armstrong and other great teachers have elaborated greatly on such facts that the greater and superior cannot and was not generated by the lesser or the inferior, showing that humans degenerated into animals, and not that animals regenerated themselves into becoming human beings. The law is the same in inorganic matter, one chemical element disintegrating into another simpler one, in which living beings depend on Biological Transmutations as Louis Kevran, Rudolf Hauschka, and other advanced scientists said debunking the chemistry and physics taught in the past.

Stevens is to be credited among those that brought to the public mind that it was grain-growing and over-grazing with cattle, sheep and goats that destroys our green earth and life thereon. Yet, considering that primates and anthropoids have degenerated from humans, as infants brought up by specific species of wild beasts prove, then Steven's affirmation about food bearing trees dating back a hundred million years, should put man's event on earth equally to that point, since it was man who selected and protected the fruit trees which he preferred for food. Wallace, quoted by Stevens said, "All the fine tropical fruits are as much cultivated productions as our apples, peaches and plums; and their wild prototype when found are generally either tasteless or inedible." The stone axe and tools were in use since prehistoric times, showing man protected his food trees and planted more from seeds for millions of years.

The Taoist wise men taught, "Far away on Mt. Ku, described as the Magical isle of the Blest, lives the ideal Heavenly man, whose skin is white as snow and he is as gentle as a young girl. He does not eat any of the five grains, but inhales air and drinks the dew. He rides on the clouds and can mount the flying dragons to wander beyond the four seas. By using spiritual power he can protect us from sickness and decay, and ensure a rich harvest", to quote Chuang Tsu. The Chinese wrote of events transpiring among their ancestors 129,000 years ago wrote Dr. P. B. Randolph. Rich harvests necessarily implies these were not of the five grains, meaning fruits and herbs were the food of their ancestors which give superior health as taught even till today by Taoist Hygienists. We have already told bout Li Chung Wan who lived 256 years on mostly herbs abstaining from meat and grains, being celebrated by the government every 50 years since his 150th year.

GENESIS OF THE HYGIENIC MOVEMENT

Natural Hygiene has and is evolving from Christian Church Theology to the original Buddhist Essene Wisdom of Jesus' Gospel as we have illustrated in our "Buddhist Essene Gospel of Jesus" as to religious doctrines. Here I have special reference as to the Law of Action, that is every Effect is produced by a corresponding Cause, visible in Nature and thus called Natural Law, or Karma engendered by our actions recent or remote. Also the Buddha taught that his precepts were based on what he himself had experienced, and not what he had heard or been taught. Thus, as disease is produced by a habit-energy pattern (Karma) contrary to Nature which gives sickness, suffering and death. The supernatural beings are the property of the priestcraft, who make man's diseases, suffering and death dependent on evil spirits possessing man, or the devil, beside its seed in the original sin. For this they reaped an abundance of animal sacrifices and other produce among the Jews, as well as tithing, churches, along with reverence and sainthood among Christians. Since Buddha dealt with Brahmins, seeking to eliminate sacrificial rites of both animals and humans, and other superstitions, gradually the converted Brahmins and those becoming monks, began to introduce satisfaction of sensual habit-energy patterns of their past needing public support by begging for cooked meals, identifying their cause by tonsural distinction, ochre robes, etc. as holymen, especially enhanced by the Jews, Christians, Taoists, and similar cults in their adoption of rituals, temples or monasteries, devils, gods, etc. Just as the Buddha did not engage in foolish talk and speculation on Brahma, God and supernatural things that they have not seen, do not know and cannot prove or experience, Natural Hygiene has evolved as Dr. Shelton explained in "Natural Hygiene, Man's Pristine Way of Life."

"It is logical to assume that in a primitive and natural state of society, normal intuition (instinct) would control the actions of the organism of man, as it does in other animals, and good health would predominate. Is it a heresy that man fully endowed in the germ to carry on the functions of living without the benefit of pedagogic warrants that he is possessed of inherent, tho now well suppressed, knowledge of life? It is thru the means of the senses and the instinctive demands of the organism that those means that pertain to organic life and development are distinguished by man. Man possesses animal appetites which he inherited along with his structure as an integral part of his organism. By this is meant that he possesses desires for food, water, activity, rest, sleep, the urge to reproduce himself, the urge to defend himself from danger or to flee from it, etc.

It is not necessary that we assume that these appetites are inherited from some ape-like ancestor. They are part of man as they are a part of all other animals, because man has the same need for them. They are expressions of the inner needs of man himself."

To this Dr. Shelton adds, "Of all animals man should be the healthiest, for he has it within his power to control the elements of his environment in his own interest and to provide himself with all the elements of a healthy existence. He has the intelligence with all his elemental needs and to apply these under all varying circumstances and conditions of life. His resources are never limited as are those of the lower animals."

The Bible Christians and early Hygienists sought the authoritative Scriptures of their time for convincing others and most often their poorly educated patients about natural laws being inviolable due to their Divine origins, and man's suffering was due to their sin, errors or violations, rather than evil spirits, since in Aramaic evil means erroneous or incorrect, and spirit refers to mind, heart or the vital principle which is life or breath. So when Jesus cast out evil spirits, it only means he freed the victims from ignorance, erroneous mind, and enlightened them on right living. The Jesus which John preached said: "Repent, the Realm of Heaven is at hand", which we slate "Change your mind, the Presence of God is right here," or within us, for God is the Way, Truth and Life. Religion should have become and is, the practice of living right, which was what the Essenes taught.

The first hygienist teacher in America was Sylvester Graham, who fortunately was not inculcated as a Medical Doctor as to the cause of disease, and seeing their failure, sought a better way. In 1840 he concluded, "When with an honest and earnest heart, I looked steadily to Nature for illumination, and with the guilelessness of a little child, give men the truth, she poured out clear and discriminating light into my soul". He was joined by Mary Gove, another empirical healer as a teacher of hygiene, who helped to let patients heal themselves by the body's self healing nature. As to Dr. Jennings, he might have gotten his clues to letting the body heal itself, from Stahl in the 17th century, who argued with considerable ability that the body had its own remedial powers, in a tradition claimed original with Hippocrates, labelled, "vix medicatrix naturae". Thus, by the added labors of Dr. Jennings, beside Dr. Trall, who joined Graham, the movement flourished. Beginning with Graham's "Journal of Health and Longevity" and Dr. R.T. Trall's "Water Cure Journal", in name only since what it taught was Hygiene, with a circulation of 18,000 in 1850, Shelton says: "So vigorous was Hygiene promulgated and so great the enthusiasm with which the people accepted it, it was estimated in January 1852 that the practitioners of the two and somewhat co-mingled schools,- Hydropathy and Hygeiotherapy,- outnumbered the practitioners of any of the medical schools, allopathic, homeopathic, eclectic and physio-medical, in this country. Whereever the Journal circulated there was invariably an improvement in Hygienic habits of the people and a corresponding decrease in fatal cases of disease and an immense saving to the people."

Sylvester Graham is the earliest Hygienist to condemn partaking of common table salt because it was an irritant and useless substance, hence a poison. By an overdose of salt it has been used to commit suicide. Similar comments explained why pepper and other spices beside sugar, that encourage one to eat what otherwise man's instincts told him was wrong. Needless to say, early Hygienists condemned food taken from animals, altho at first Graham allowed milk. However, it was Graham who called attention to eating whole-grains, rye, barley and wheat or corn bread, and altho he called them Graham bread, or Graham crackers made with honey, this is the only way one hears his name, except among Health literature. Potatoes with Jerusalem artichokes were classified as fruits, rather than roots. One wonders what fresh fruits and vegetables Graham ate at Boston, except in the summer and fall, since he was before the modern rapid transportation, refrigeration, which made such foods available from the south. Also, strict raw food eaters growing their own food, use carrots, mild turnips, rutabaga, kohlrabi, sprouted sunflower, legumes, etc. that in his restrictions and times were little known.

Now, Graham and Hygienists were not original nor unique as to ideas on certain foods. In Yoga, food is classified by the Gunas, that is three kinds: Sattwic or pure, Rajasic or exciting or irritating, and Tamasic which make one dull and stupid. To quote Swami Sivananda, "As is the food so is the mind. The mind is made out of the subtle portion of food. Food exercises tremendous influence on the mind. Fish, meat, garlic and onions, excite passions. They are Rajasic and Tamasic. You can get food nutrition and energy form fruit, vegetables, milk, almonds, gram, dhall. Those who eat meat have a crematorium in their stomachs. They are unfit for Yogic practices and spiritual contemplation. Excess salt in the blood produces a dry sort of itch, thirst, constipation, inability to bear the sun's heat and headache". (Samadhi Yoga) Elsewhere vegetables above the ground are recommended as sun foods, and below the ground are more tamasic, low, earthy or dull the mind comparatively. Of course, these Yogis were not exemplary in health, often with a big paunch, yet they did make keen observations as to diet, outside their excess use of cooked foods, legumes, rice, etc.

Writing March 6th, 1834 in his "Esculapian Tablets", Sylvester Graham said: "With the universal opinion that all their disease and suffering are the direct and arbitrary and even vindictive influence of their God, or gods, mankind has cherished no other fear of disease than that which grows out of their gross superstitions- fear that God would send sickness and death upon them, independently of any laws which he had established in health and disease. Therefore, as a general truth, it never occurred to them that there is any relation between their own voluntary habits, customs and indulgences, and disease with which they were afflicted. Consequently they have never sought to find the causes of disease within the precincts of voluntary conduct and have never taken any care to prevent disease by avoiding causes. The whole drift therefore of the human world in all generations has been to one point, on this subject,- the ascertainment of remedies for diseases of every form."

Altho the tomato was eaten by the Indians, the Europeans believed it was poisonous, and thus medicinally used as a substitute for calomel, uniquely to the good in errors. Graham began teaching it was good food, valuable like apples and other fresh fruits. The first new advocates of vegetarianism were called Pythagoreans, but then it became Grahamism. Even in our times, the Merc Manual of Materia Medica among hundreds of prescription drugs, there is rare mention of the Gerson diet of fruits and vegetables as a treatment along with their drugs, seeking to obliterate Graham and early Hygienists from medical knowledge.

One of the things that Vitalogical Healing and Hygiene sought to reform of the Hygienic System is to point to the fact that fruit with nuts preached by past advocates, specifically gives a desire to drink earth water from springs, ponds, etc. Hygienists claim all inorganic substances are poisonous, or pathological, making this one inconsistent exception. Yet, inorganic water from wells or springs is laden with lime, iron oxide, salt, etc. beside being without life itself, causing a coating to form in kettles beside water containers. If only succulent vegetables and juicy fruits are eaten, without the driest of all foods, nuts such as walnuts with 2% water, almonds 5% and pinions 3%, there is no calling for nuts, grains or legumes, since all the organic minerals, vitamins, enzymes and amino acids needed for health are found in green leafy vegetables and fruits that give the needed carbohydrates by choice of fruits.

Past Hygienists believed men should reproduce like animals by instinct, not realizing this instinct originated in seminal substances they were eating, haphazardly breeding children who due to worldly environment, thus they rebelled, ate meat, etc. The food aid sent to starving nations has been grains, more reproductive substance, that did not solve the problem, but reproduced more of it. William Lamb, M.D. practicing in England, argued man was not equipped anatomically for drinking from streams or ponds, and many animals never drink. So in the Journal, Graham, said this might be so if the proportion of fluid and solids in food eaten in a physiologically correct diet was in proportion to the fluid and solids in the body. We have shown already that the primate anthropoids were not provided with nuts, eating exclusively of fruits and greens. Apes have no exotic theories about above ground leafy greens and fruits. Rodents like squirrels, pack rats, etc. hoard nuts from trees for the winter, in the summer invading my garden to feast on vegetables in California. Shall we thus classify man as a rodent? Hygienists believing in use of nuts seemed to argue in this cause. What fresh fruit and vegetables did Graham eat in winter when summer fruits were gone? Thus, the heavy reliance on dead inorganic water, up to 95% if one was an exclusive nutarian, which is fine for rodents, and likewise the rodent over-population which in confined areas leads to cannibalism, similar to overfeeding of hens on grains. This seed based diet causes wars, feeds soldiers, and is in conquest of grain-growing land, more than flesh-eating often.

However, Graham did concede that there is a need for bulk in the diet. Moreover, nut kernels contain poisonous skins as found in the almond, walnuts, and cashew nuts which have to be blanched, and oleaginous seeds as Dr. T. de la Torre recommends has tannic acid coating, showing Nature's argument, protecting them for becoming a basic diet, and thus giving indigestion from toxic reaction. But man again thinks he can evade Nature, just as he did refining grains, degerming grains, just like his need to spay or castrate humans or animals pacifying them. On the walls of the intestines are villi which take in the amino acids, vitamins, minerals, enzymes that are held in the blood and tissues to do the work of life, but various Hygienic authors have suggested that tannic acid, and similar food poisons need to be removed so one does not harm these sensitive tissues, debilitating the lacto-bacterial functions, just as antibiotics cripple them giving a need for curds from milk, sourkraut, etc.

Also, in his "Esculapian Tablets" of 1834, Graham wrote: "Disease never results from constitutional and legitimate operation of the human system. Every such operation is health and only health"; in brief he points out that disease is the disturbance of that process by an offending cause, and thus to correct this one needs to restore the human system into healthy operation, and not adding further causes to the disorder called disease. For this, living strictly for health is necessary, not by partial observation, but an integral natural way of health. Only man is capable of this, since even apes suffer with runny noses and were heard coughing, squirrels and other such animals of the wilds are filled with worms and parasites, etc., showing that nature is only perfect so long as sentient beings

conform to her laws, which man is best equipped to do, altho he continues to ignore this wisdom just as great men have taught. Prior to Graham,
mankind seems to have accepted disease as a normal substance.

In general all are agreed that narcotics, tea, coffee, colas, cocoa or chocolate, tobacco, alcohol, marijuana, etc. do not constitute good food for
health at meals. However when it comes to salads, Hygienists are not
very liberal as to salad dressing of any kind, insisting food not palatable
alone should not be eaten until one gets a natural appetite for them. Dr.
Trall said "Olive oil is not recommended as necessary or useful, but as
preferable to lard or butter. We do not teach nor believe in greasing food
in any manner, nor of shortening it in any degree". Well, the way he puts
it, that food should not be greased, or oiled to get it down, does sound
reasonable. Your author spent a good part of his early life in Ecuador
without funds, and thus used potatoes with vegetable salad, or where
bananas, avocados or tomatoes were available, he relished with the salads. However, due to poisoning with pesticides, with inability to digest
anything, he ended up using cottage cheese or curds, and clabber with
salads, replenishing the lacto-bacteria for intestinal assimilation. Avocado
or tomato served well when available without poisonous chemical treatment.

In Orthotrophy Vol. II of The Hygienic System, Dr. Shelton gives various vegetable salads in correct combining with lettuce, cabbage, celery,
carrots, endive, green peppers, etc. in menus that include either avocados or tomatoes, or cucumber or onions as ideal diet. For beginning the
Reform Diet he allows avocados, baked potato, nuts, wholegrain bread,
cottage cheese, various steamed vegetables, baked squash, fresh corn
alone with two or three vegetables raw. However, altho the apes did not
mix nor fix themselves salads, they took their wild celery, nettles, borage,
banana plant pith, as they came, letting the digestion mix them with their
fruits indiscriminately. But, "A clear mucous ran from their noses and
an explosive cough interrupted the jungle stillness. Respiratory troubles
are the principle causes of death in gorillas. In captivity they die easily of
pneumonia. They also die of roundworm, resembling hookworms, intestinal parasites and chronic diarrhea". Thus, the encyclopedia Britannica
research team did not find the gorilla with all this powerful build a health
example of Primates, possibly due to nearly exclusive wild salads, with 2
to 15% fruit only. The other primates did better, 50 to 67% fruit with their
greens, being more appropriate. That they should have runny noses this
your author found true when he ate extra bananas, in the tropical climates due to asphysxia not being able to oxidize the carbohydrates while
in the temperate climate like that of Quito, he could live on bananas alone
when he could not afford other fruits, so this proves the banana chemistry

in plant and fruit was the offending factor. In his "Cookbook" (1854), Dr. Trall says seasoning herbs, such as sage, thyme, the mints, dill, fennel, tansy, tarragon, nasturtium, chervil, rosemary, lavender, basil, angelica, anise, cumin, etc. can hardly be classed as food. True, one would not care to live on any or any mixture alone. Then he attacks, mushrooms, ferns and lichens. The primates do relish ferns, mushrooms being growths without sunlight can be suspicioned and often are poisonous. Onions, garlic, leeks, shallots, chives, radishes, watercress and mustard contain mustard oil and other highly irritating substances. However, in his Orthotrophy, Shelton allows sweet onions, scallions, radishes, watercress, the watercress and hot radishes being especially hard on your author's kidneys.

A physician writing in the British Medical Journal, pointed out that mustard, taken with food is more harmful to the stomach than aspirin and may occasion more bleeding than the drug. Some varieties of onions are as piquant as mustard, as are also certain varieties of radishes, such as large white radishes, the large black radish and the horseradish. Shelton believes because they are so acrid they are probably indigestible, and includes water cress and hot cabbages in the list.

Trall was of the opinion that salt (sodium chloride) was worst than useless, the "free use of salt irritates the mouth, throat and stomach, causing thirst and fever, and provokes an unnatural appetite, while it loads the circulating fluids with foreign ingredients which the excretory organs must labor inordinately to get rid of". It causes the excess intake of water that bloats the body, putting on extra weight of no value in what is called edema. The reason it increases the flow of saliva, gastric juice and mucous is because it is an irritating substance, like other condiments, which seek to lessen the irritation by diluting it with liquids.

Next, Dr. Trall says that vinegar, sourkraut and similar decomposed products are unfit for food. Shelton compares the fermentation of hog's swill barrel to kraut. They ignore the use of yogurt, curds or buttermilk in cases of longevity, as promoted by French chemist M. Roberts and Metchnikoff, as did Bodansky's Physiological Chemistry of 1903. Now according to French physiologist, Claude Bernard, glycogen is stored in the muscles and used in muscular activity. A man running in a tread mill, breathing pure oxygen, increased the lactic acid content from 20 mg. per 100 cc. of blood to 86 mg. In turn breathing air, running twice as fast the lactic acid rose from 8.5 to 204 milligram per 100 cubic centimeters of blood. After entering the blood a portion of the lactic acid is excreted in the urine, which increases with violent exercise. But another part is returned to the liver, there to be resynthesized into glycogen. An excess in glycosuria and hypoglycemia, as in your author's inability to oxidize carbohydrates of bananas in low altitudes due to asphyxia, thus burdens the kidneys with excess lactic acid. This points to why Yogis in India use curds, and Westerners find cottage cheese, the whey removing must of the objectionable lactic acid, but not so necessary in cold climates. Graham and Trall both thought fresh milk and cream preferable to butter or curds, but rejected them to be consistent with doctrine against animal products of any kind, not realizing that fresh milk is the cause of nasal catarrh of their findings, and that predigested curds or cottage cheese as it is called in the west, is more assimilable.

Avocados, dried olives, like the curds do not grease or oil one's food to get it down, any more than oily nuts and seeds, yet the tablespoon of olive, sesame, sunflower, etc. oil with a large salad surely is not prone to this objection. Our point is that the human system was never programmed for nut and seed consumption, like those of rodents. There is more in life than reproduction, population and pollution problems. Shelton especially was against characterizing Hygiene as a "spiritual" movement, yet insisted it was all-inclusive, which would be a sad fate for something that started out as moral and a higher spiritual way of life once under the Banner of Bible Christians.

Laws, including natural laws certainly are not to be characterized as material which identifies with the ever-changing and evanescent and the illusory as the Buddha characterized them. Only spiritual laws are eternal, permanent and dependable as the guide in life, whether this be of a physical or spiritual nature, or what we call Nature itself and consequently man is a spiritual being, himself, when he becomes a conscious believer in the Eternal rather than the Evanescent.

Nor did Hygiene start as pure Hygiene as a movement, coming as one might vulgarly state it, as riding piggy-back on often related parts, until the special name was invented resting on the Greek goddess Hygeia, again spiritual in nature, just as Jesus characterized man as "Ye are Gods". Sylvester Graham, who was not a physician, was pre-eminently the father of the philosophy of physiology, and a group of Graham's students founded the world's first physiological society, "The American Physiological Society" in 1837 at Boston before the term Hygiene was coined. They established the "Graham Journal of Health and Longevity", the "Library of the American Physiological Society" and the world's first Health Food Store, and even attempted to start a Physiological Infirmary, giving physiological care for the sick without drugs. Mary Gove joined Graham founding female divisions of the Society which with both groups of men and women held the "American Health Convention", held meetings in Boston in 1838, in New York in 1839, later even in Ohio.

In turn, as we have seen Dr. Russell T. Trall published in 1851 his "Hy-dropathic Encyclopedia", which was derived from European Water Cure systems, which he systemized as a Healing Art based entirely on Hygien-ic principles, in 1862 forming the National Hygienic Association. To char-acterize Dr. Trall as a Hydropath, because he first studied and wrote on Hydropathy, is like calling Martin Luther Roman Catholic because he first initiated his career as a Catholic. His Journal also started as the "Water Cure Journal", and even after fully accepting Hygiene fully, and claimed water had no power whatever in curing disease, still his "Hygeio-Ther-apeutic College" was founded on the basis of Hygienic Medication and other misleading medical terms.

In turn, Isaac Jennings was a medical practitioner who after 20 years lost all confidence in drugging and bleeding, to rely entirely thereafter on Hygienic care which was so successful that he was honored with an honorary degree by Yale University. Since he revealed his secret using only placebo medicines, many turned against him as fraudulent, but that is like charging Jesus Christ of the Gospels, as being a fake because he taught fasting and prayer, or even rubbed spittle in a man's eyes, or com-manded them to take up their bed and walk. Such a system as Dr. Jen-nings practices has always been called faith or spiritual healing. With his success with such a "do-nothing medication", and learning of Graham's physiological system as "Orthopathy" which is described as "relying solely upon the healing powers of the body and placing his patients in the best possible conditions for the operation of the body's own healing pro-cesses, by means of rest, fasting, diet, pure air and other Hygienic factors, he permitted his patients to get well", as quoted from Shelton's "Natural Hygiene".

In Dr. Jennings first book "Medical Reform" published in 1847 he ex-plained his THEORY OF HUMAN LIFE. In his day, life and living were scientifically based on chemical action and materialism. In turn Jennings joined the vitalists, using words like vitality, vital force in place of Life in Latin terms for the vital principle and Nature. "Human Life consists in or results from the union of the principle, denominated the vital or living principle, with matter curiously and wonderfully wrought into a system of organs, originally, by the fiat of the Almighty, and continued and propagated by a self-preserving and self perpetuating faculty. Of the particular nature or essence of this vital principle,- how it is applied, or how it operates in exciting motion,- we know nothing. We can only judge of it from its operations and effects, its sensible manifestations.

I:- This principle, and this alone, produces, sustains and controls all vital action in man, whether perfect or imperfect. No other principle, power or force can supply its place, and perform living action in its stead. When this is present, there is life, when it is exhausted, death ensues.

II:- Life results as naturally from the presence of the vital principle as water runs down a hill, and the former is no more a forced state than the later. Nor can the inorganic affinities, such as fermentation, decomposition or putrefaction play upon matter charged with the vital principle.

III:- In whatever way the vital energy is furnished, whether dispensed from an unreplenishable fund, deposited at the commencement of life in a given amount to some portion of the brain,- or transmitted directly from Deity,- or in whatever way, or from whatever source it is furnished, it becomes available present, there is life, when it is exhausted, death ensues.

II:- Life results as naturally from the presence of the vital principle as water runs down a hill, and the former is no more a forced state than the later. Nor can the inorganic affinities, such as fermentation, decomposition or putrefaction play upon matter charged with the vital principle.

III:- In whatever way the vital energy is furnished, whether dispensed from an unreplenishable fund, deposited at the commencement of life in a given amount to some portion of the brain,- or transmitted directly from Deity,- or in whatever way, or from whatever source it is furnished, it becomes available by the distributing organs, in a regular income, at a greater or lesser rate, and at all times and under all circumstances, till the supply ceases.

IV: It was evidently the design of the Creator of man's physical system, that there should be at all times a large supply of vital energy in store, over and above the income, or what was required for ordinary current expenditure, ready for any emergency, that a sudden and extraordinary draft upon it might not produce bankruptcy.

V:- The production or income of the vital principle can, by no human possibility, be increased,- its expenditure, general and local, may be accelerated.

VI:- The vital energy can never be in excess, yet the best economy of life demands that it should be used freely when the supply in store will admit it, especially in childhood and youth. It requires less power to sustain the different functions of life when the organs are well developed and in sound condition, than when they are not; it is good economy, therefore, to expend power enough on the muscles of voluntary motion to give extension and tone to the whole system.

VII: The seat or depository of this power is the brain, and most probable, each tissue of working agents or acting organs, by and thru which power is expended, has a separate depository of power for the supply of its own wants, which may be called individual depository.

At the head of the great sympathetic nerve is a large depository for power destined to act as a reserve supply or balancing power, to afford succor to any feeble oppressed organ that may need special relief; and particularly to guard and sustain those organs that are essential to life. This may be called the general or common depository. The ganglions or little brains, formed by the convolutions of nerves, and found in every part of the body, in the vicinity of every organ, proportioned in size and importance of the organ, also serve as sub-reservoirs or special depositories of power, to act on the spur of occasion, and furnish aid to their respective wards, in periods of sudden danger, before help could reach them from headquarters. The vital current is, moreover, not subject to a retrograde motion; but when the power leaves its depository it keeps its own proper channel till it reaches its place of destination, and is then used. And lastly, the vital energy is not transferable or interchangeable by or between the individual organs or their depositories; on the contrary the only source of aid of feeble organs, beyond their own fountains of strength, is in the common depository of power.

VIII:- By virtue of a law to be noticed presently, and more elucidated in sequel, the vital energy is transmitted from the repositories to the several parts of the organism thru the medium of the nerves, as circumstances require, or according to the necessities of the system and ability to supply. The power may be with held from some parts and appropriated to others, or held in check for replenishment, and thus become latent, leaving the parts from which it has been withheld, for the time being, unable to act.

IX: When the vital energy abounds in ample quantity, in a well developed and sound state of the organism, the depositories all full and overflowing, and there is nothing to prevent a free distribution of the energy or impede the actions of the organ, every part of the system will be supplied with the power to the utmost necessity, and every function will be performed with promptness, ease and vigor. If blood be drawn from the body under these circumstances, it will exhibit a lively, florid, healthy appearance, and long resist the law of decomposition. Wounds and bruises also heal readily, and physical good feeling, animation and universal symptoms of health and strength prevail. But when there is great deficiency of this power, it will be indicated by symptoms or appearances opposite to those just enumerated modified by the circumstances. Yet the power still remaining, be it more or less, will be appropriated according to the necessities of the whole system; first to its present safety; and when this is secured, to its future welfare and prolongation of life.

X:- This vital principle, which generates the living fiber, and produces and controls its action, is itself under law,- a law which is fixed and uniform in its operations as the law of gravitation, or any physical law. The tendency of all its motions, is in one direction, towards the point of perfect health, and that to with all its force. Finally, from the foregoing may be deduced the following:

GENERAL CONCLUSIONS

When there is a perfect organization and structure, a full supply of vital power, and nothing to impede or disturb its operations, there will be perfect health. When the organic structure is defective the vital energy deficient, or an impeding and disturbing cause present, health will be defective or impaired. The kind and degree of impaired action will depend on the nature of the part affected, the nature and extent of the part affected, the degree of deficiency of vital power and the amount of force exerted by the impeding or disturbing causes. The process by which recovery is to be effected when there is structural derangement or defect, may be called a repairing process. When there is simply a deficiency of power, it may be called a recruiting process. Both of these are the work of nature,- vital work. Art may serve as a hand-maid to nature in this work by removing causes, when they are present and can be removed at a less expense of vital energy and less injury to organs by art than they can be by nature,- by furnishing nature with suitable material for carrying on her work,- and in general providing that entire condition of body and mind and kept favorable to the restorative process. But the repairing and recruiting are nature's own work, in which art can have no share."

OUR COMMENTARY:

When a junior in high school (1936), I had been a vegetarian for over a year, read old Physical Culture magazines and Dr. Lust's "Natures Path", etc. and received chiropractic adjustments in Seattle as an experiment. Then, the old book shop yielded and old copy of "Principles and Practice" by Dr. D.D. Palmer on the Philosophy of Chiropractic. Reading Dr. Jennings above treatise, it brought back memories of Palmer's presentation. Dr. Shelton suggests that vitality, vital energy and vital force above mentioned should be replaced with nerve energy, nervous influence and nerve impulse. While Palmer made use of structural defects cutting off the full supply of vital power to justify spinal adjustments, Dr. Jennings intended this to be achieved by fasting, and all the elements of a healthy life.

Dr. Isaac Jennings was the first to make professional use of the fast in sickness in America starting in 1822. Eight years later Sylvester Graham also advocated it. Where did Jennings get it? The Bible Christians, who established themselves in America 5 years before 1822, Jennings conversion, may have preached it along with vegetarianism and eschewing alcoholic beverages, tobacco, and other narcotics. If not, due to his conscience in using drugs killing people, and decision to avoid such treatment, he probably read his Bible and prayed for a better solution. In my old Rheims-Challoner version, John the Baptist preached saying, "Do penance for the kingdom of heaven is at hand" (Mt.3:2) "I indeed baptize with water unto penance" (3:11) And every where later versions say repentance instead of penance, but, the Aramaic term here means, repent, change the mind, turn back, vomited, regurgitate or refuse food. Our Rheims version has footnote insisting this is to punish past sins by fasting and prayer. "They that are in health need not a physician, but they that are ill. Go then and learn this meaning, I will have mercy and not sacrifice. I am not come to call the just but sinners. Then came to him the disciples of John, saying, Why do we and the Pharisees fast often, but thy disciples do not fast? And Jesus said to them, Can the children of the bridegroom mourn, as long as the bridegroom is with them? But the day will come, when the bridegroom shall be taken away from them; then they shall fast". (Mt.9:12-15) The footnote interprets 9:15 as: friends or companions.

In Matthew 17:18 says: "Then came the disciples to Jesus secretly and said: Why could we not cast him out? Jesus said unto them: Because of your unbelief. For, amen I say to you, if you have faith as a grain of mustard seed, you shall say to the mountain, remove from hence hither, and it shall remove: nothing shall be impossible to you. But this kind is not cast out but by prayer and fasting". This proves that Jesus fasted 40 days and nights (4:2) to get the "power to move mountains", confirmed by Luke 4:14, "And Jesus returned in the power of the Spirit into Galilee" after the fast. Mark repeats the question of disciples as to why they could not cast out the devil or evil spirit of error in 9:28 saying, "This kind can go out by nothing but by fasting and prayer".

He did not expect the victim to fast, but rather he referred to his 40 day fast giving him such spiritual power. In Luke 13:3,5 he likewise says: "But unless you do penance you shall likewise perish." In the table of references, it also says Matthew 9:15 means "Fasting is to be observed by all the children of Christ". Thus Bishop Challoner's Rheims version was in strict agreement with Thomas Aquinas theology of the Hypostasis of the Word and Son of God, and proven also by the fact that Mark 1:4 says: "John was in the desert baptizing and preaching the baptism of penance unto remission of sins". But then in 1:15 he says the Christ did not include fasting and prayer, that is, penance in his preaching to converts saying: "The kingdom of God is at hand: repent and believe in the gospel". Thus, the son of Simon Peter, who is only the political Christ or Messiah, that was crucified, shows he differs in the doctrine that is preached by the Evangelist John, Matthew and Luke, that only faith derived from fasting and prayer like he practices for 40 days was required of all the disciples or children of Christ.

What my point is in showing that Protestant versions of the Bible completely ignore the use of the word "Penance" meaning fasting and prayer, while these early Catholic versions like that of Bishop Challoner emphasized it with footnotes even. Protestants held that faith and repentance were good enough, but thus they never could achieve sainthood. The first Apostles under James, Bishop of Jerusalem, laid emphasis on works, which made ones faith valid. So what makes it important is that the Crucifixion of Simon only made him King of the Jews as "Jesus Bar-Abbas", son of famous Zealot criminal politically, but "I say to you, that there shall be joy in heaven upon one sinner that does penance, more than ninety-nine just who need not penance". Luke 15:7 here is repeated in 15:10. So when John is emphasized as the person or hypostasis of the Word or Son of God in speaking the words preached by Jesus as our Lord, it means his insistence on works gave him power of miracles and glory in heaven. When Jesus was asked, by what authority he did things, he inferred that his power came after his 40 day fast, henceforth speaking as the very person of the spiritual Saviour. "The baptism of John, whence was it? From heaven or from men?" Power and authority in Aramaic are synonymous. Thus it is sainthood or glory in heaven that is gained by works.

Thus, I have had to give a detailed explanation, which the letter Hygienist knew nothing about, without such a theological background. Dr. Isaac Jennings certainly must have found this elaborate promotion of fasting to develop faith and self-healing power, which means "let alone" or "do nothing" since the body heals itself and physicians are given the credit. After his first step in lustration or "baptism" of penance, or fasting and prayer, Jesus gave us the sustenance of "Living Water" and "Living Bread" or live uncooked food as the requirement of Salvation or Life Everlasting. (Jn.6:51)

However, let us not just reiterate the whole healing philosophy of John the Baptist, Apostle and Evangelist (one person) who preached the Word or Son of God's "Buddhist Essene Gospel of Jesus", since it may best obtained reading our Aramaic translation with an intrinsical understanding of the subject. Sufficient is the self-evident fact that Jennings, Graham and Trall had intuitively picked up the thought patterns from this powerful dynamo among the First Followers of our Lord and Savior's teaching while reading their Bibles. Whatever the actual source of the translation of the Bibles it must have resembled the author's first Catholic New Testament text, before his later studies of the originals in the Syriac dialect of Aramaic.

An even more venturesome explanation would be to hazard a guess Isaac Jennings, M.D., had studied Latin at medical studies in school as required in our day to be able the name plants and other substance by their obscure Latin term, and since the most available text for a study of the language was the Latin Vulgate version of the Bible of Jerome of the 4th Century, this lead him to uncover the true Natural Hygienic factors of what he called "Orthopathy, or Right Treatment". They still make use of meaning with T.L.C. in prescription in modern hospitals, but instead of Tender Loving Care, they practice the opposite with shots, transfusions, pills at all hours, exploratory surgery and hundreds of other disagreeable or torturous ordeals as routine. Since Allopathic Medicine, the art of treating or curing disease is focused on disease, the least could be hoped for true health of humans by studying such a misnomer for such a "science".

"The Materia Hygienica compromises all the elements of nature which have a physiological relation to the human constitution; they are those elements most intimately concerned with the phenomena of life,- with development, growth, maintenance, repair, healing and reproduction. To state this differently, Hygienic means are those things which are used by the organism in the normal functioning processes,- light, air, food, water, temperature, activity, rest, sleep, cleanliness, emotional poise, etc. These means are classed as Hygienic because they relate to the preservation of health." (Dr. Shelton) He continues: "Physicians would have us believe that the needs of the sick organism are extraordinary, exotic and rare, requiring great skill in their administration, and that they are such unusual efficaciousness that only the highly trained expert can be entrusted with their administration. As Hygienists, we contend, on the other hand, that remedies in any true sense are those materials or influences which supply physiological needs, either of materials or of conditions that are favorable to the operations of the powers inherent in the living organism or that remove the causes of disease and which are not chemically or physiologically incompatible with the structures and functions of life."

THE MATERIA MEDICA OF MODERN QUACKERY TODAY IN OFFICIALDOM AND THE RENAISSANCE OF NATURAL VITALOGICAL HYGIENE FORESEEN

We found as the definition of "Alchemy" in Webster's dictionary is given as: (1) "The medical chemical science, the great objects of which were to change base metals into gold, and to discover the universal cure for disease and the means of infinitely prolonging life. (2) A method or power of transmutation, seemingly miraculous change of one thing into another." In nature this is being done in biological Transmutations but this is dangerous for man as seen in nuclear research or not for men to attempt or to proffer in doing. However, our theme now is Modern Quackery. Among the greatest contributors to this chemical science was Paracelsus (1493-1541) at a time when the discovery of a New World was found in America, and Chemotherapy began to be practiced. The books of such Alchemy purport cinnabar as the universal alkahest, or the "universal solvent". Cinnabar is defined as (1) Red mercuric sulfide HgS, the only important ore of mercury; (2) Artificial red mercuric sulfide used as a pigment; (3) The color vermilion.

Next, Mercury is defined as (1) Roman god identified with Hermes, the messenger of gods, the god of commerce, manual skill, eloquence, cleverness, travel and thievery. From this is derived "Merx" or merchandise, and thus today physicians often use the Merc Manual of Materia Medica to prescribe their chemotherapeutic Rx (Recipe) of pharmaceutical merchandise. But here by mercury we refer also to a heavy, silver white metallic element, liquid at ordinary temperature, which sometimes occurs in a free state but usually in combination with sulfur, quick-silver. The common term "quick silver" generated the great store of mythical medical superstitions about what it is and does. Obviously, the word was allegorical in this since "quick" means living, revived from the dead, or transmuted, so as to give curative power, but "quick" also means fast, so that the Alchemists achieved as "quick silver" or fast silver or gold for their marvellous claims purported for cinnabar and mercurial chemistry.

As to "quackery", the "Quacks" were the users of "Quack salver", which is Dutch and German for quick silver, in English even seeming to imply saviour or salvation, while the definition thus alluded for "quack" is a "boastful pretender to medical skill, a person dishonestly claiming to effect a cure." Thus the art of fast money, silver, merchandising and thievery in the use of chemotherapeutic medicines is the real Quack. Now, at the time of the Hygienists Jennings, Graham and Trall, the great alkahest was Camomel, or mercurous chloride. The Merc Manual still lists it because of "its reaction with proteins in the cells of an organism it is a virulent poison". A very dilute solution (1:1,000) is used as an antiseptic. It is used in fevers, largely for its alleged purgative action, but also because it was said to act on the liver.

Its use, as well as the use of all mercurials (Merc lists 17) results in bone necrosis, destruction of the glands, gumma of the arteries, growths of syphilitic origin, severe impairment of the nervous system, etc. Earlier we have cited claims by physicians providing for a lifetime practice by prescribing camomile for various kinds of fever, so as to suppress the body's own healing action in cleansing the body of its toxins, or other complaints, since the side-effects of its poisoning generated such a lucrative quick silver business. As with the case of gumma, they produce a third stage of syphilis with their mercurials, and then treated the mercury-caused disease with their mercurials, and then treated the mercury-caused disease with more mercury. The result was claimed, "Once a syphilitic, always a syphilitic", showing just how such poisons provide for a fast quack merchants fortune. Mercury is another protoplasmic poison, qualified as an antibiotic being destructive to all forms of life. All this began due to the myth of living silver attributes, supposedly giving life and reviving patients.

Pharmaco-dynamics are in reality bio-dynamics, in the case of such poisons, drugs, cannot act or cure and do anything fraudulently attributed to them by chemotherapy. The substance is inert, dead, but being such virulent poisons, the body acts on them seeking to eliminate them but fails, since they kill the biological or physiological living protoplasm that they come in contact with, destroying the body's power to act.

We have described the scene as it appeared well over a century and a half ago, but with the modern era of wonder drugs in the midst of the 20th century, all that has been changed is the names of the poisonous drugs of the merx merchants. As John in his Apocalypse tells it: "The merchants of earth shall weep and mourn over her, for no man shall buy their merchandise anymore... for the merchants have been the great men of earth, for all the nations have been deceived by thy enchantments", Since here at the end of the Second Millennium we have witnessed the abandoning of medical methods of poisoning and surgery with more and more doctors turning to alternate methods of edication and treatment.

Chief among the wonder drugs in claims of miracles performed was a terrific poison, altho even claimed to rank with folklore medicines, as bread mold, was Penicillin, which derived its popularity becuse it was less lethal than camomile. So taking into account the great mortality and drug-caused diseases produced by camomel, the use of Penicillin produced less drug-caused diseases and mortality, so the greater amount of patients surviving its so-called therapy was now credited to having been cured by it. Just as in the case of your author, one drugless practitioner proclaimed that I was too healthy due to my fasting, natural diet and life to be killed by even such super-poisons. Sir Alexander Fleming, the supposed discoverer of Penicillin, was given the Nobel Prize for it in 1945, being thus accounted among "the great men of earth" in its lauded "enchantments" of saving so many lives simply because it did not sacrifice as many lives, altho still with millions dying from its use. The same has been purported for nuclear medicines, operations cutting out vital organs, and other such miraculous or heroic cures.

Why was penicillin claimed to be good? (1) Disease is due to the invasion of the body by microorganisms. (2) Penicillin kills micro-organisms. (3) Penicillin is selective in its killing, killing microorganisms only and not the microscopic cells of the body. (4) After the invading germs are killed off, the diseased tissue heals rapidly. (They are not really healed by penicillin, which is a poison, but by something else.) (5) It is possible to give enough penicillin to kill millions of bacteria without seriously damaging or killing the patient.

But today physicians are of the opinion that this treatment now has serious drawbacks. When too little is given the remaining organisms revive and the infection goes on from where it left off. Greater doses result in some of these organisms developing resistance to the antibiotic. Then the physician has to switch to another drug, or let the disease follow its natural course. Such is the medical method of exorcism, casting out the microscopic devils, that the ordinary vision cannot see. So now penicillin is claimed good for minor ailments and stronger poisons are allegedly needed for serious infections. What more, the patient may develop an allergy to the drug. Beside it is not effective with some microorganisms including viruses, such as which cause the common cold. All these excuses are given to avoid the confession that this antibiotic is not the remedy but rather a killer and crippler of fallacious pretensions. Yet five hundred tons of penicillin in its time were prescribed every year, often indiscriminately.

Before penicillin almost everyone with streptococcal infections of the blood died, 9 in 10 with meningococcic meningitis failed to live. One out of three victims of pneumococcic pneumonia died. Now-a-days almost all of these patients live. These supposed facts were quoted in the "Daily News" of New York. But why did the patients die before the use of penicillin? This, these sources did not dare to reveal. Did they die of the disease, or of the treatment in vogue? These informants never investigate the death rate in these diseases among those not treated by drugs. So the only evidence of "curing" of diseases, is that the medical profession changes from a lethal mode of treatment, to one that is less lethal, and interprets the fewer deaths as meaning that a new drug cures patients. By interpreting the abandoning of mercurials and iodide of potassium that were formerly employed in the treatment of syphilis, the newer drugs get their fame from killing less people or a greater survival rate. Thus the fame of penicillin rests on the fact it killed less people, altho crippling the survivors, who now are chronic invalids.

The so-called allergy to penicillin is a cover-up to hide the body's resistance seeking to defend itself form the administered poison. There is no harmless poison. Next came Neutrapem, a poison to fight a poison, and so on, which again have unpredictable side effects. Drugs of the strep-tomycin family, including kanamycin are a threat to one's hearing. The medics shrug this off, saying they must take protective measures seeing an informed physician. But there are no warning signs that precede the destruction of the blood's cells with chloramphenicol. Dr. Herbert Shelton whose Hygienic Review we follow in these assertions, adds that only a hardened criminal will continue to administer a drug that destroys the red blood cells and produces anemia in infants.

New York specialists discontinued using penicillin in disease because they had so many deaths in their practice from such causes. So H.T. Hyman, M.D. advises his readers to be careful with medications. He tells of three murders: (1) A 30 year old woman with inflammation of the pelvic organs; (2) a 65 year old woman who has a cold for 10 days (3) a 21 year old woman in the 8th week of pregnancy complicated by pain in the appendix region. Each one of them were given a shot of penicillin, altho none had anything seriously wrong with them. They were not in the slightest danger, but all were killed. All these could have been saved by Hygienic means. Dr. Hyman insists, "All three might still be alive, and a new baby been born had they received thoughtful care and at the most, a dose of penicillin given by the mouth. Some physicians advise a sensitiv-ity test before giving penicillin orally." What is being said is "let alone", "do nothing" care is the best treatment after all.

We are going to quote more taken from Dr. H.M. Shelton's book, "Health for the Millions": "Physicians derive most of their income from disease, not from health. Health would be their undoing. The hospital industry is at present the fifth largest industry in the country. Health would close the doors of hospitals and stop the wheels of pharmaceutical industries. These men and their institutions have a vested interest in sickness, hence their promotion of immunization schemes, which while they do not im-munize, do produce disease, and the selling of cures, many of which are productive of worse diseases than the ones for which they were given."

Testifying before a Senate Subcommittees in 1967, Leighton E. Cuff M.D. professor of medicine at the University of Florida stated that "the adverse effect of non-prescription drugs, as well as prescription drugs is responsi-ble for the hospitalization and deaths of a significant number of patients. Testifying before the same Subcommittees in 1968, were three fathers, two of them physicians, who told of the deaths of their three children as the result of being treated with chloromycitin. A common result of the administration of this drug is aplastic anemia, an iatrogenic disease that usually proves fatal". The bone marrow pathology cripples and destroys the body's ability to make red corpuscles. "The drugging system as it increases in toxicity, floods the world with adverse side effects, iatrogenic diseases and deaths from so-called allergic reactions, but this does not deter physicians in their prescribing practices. Neither does it prevent the continued manufacture of drugs, nor stop the search for new and more poisonous ones. They resent any activity that interferes with their profits from drugs."

"After 2.500 years of intensive farming of the drug idea, we are reduced to this: we cannot tell in advance of prescribing a drug what effect will follow in a given case or in a given condition except that we know that every drug is a poison and produces disease."

We have quoted these provocative statements from Shelton's book to compel the reader to investigate for himself studying his books and even conservative views for those skeptics which are hard fixed in old beliefs by looking into the Alternative Medical Association, and a growing dissention among physicians today so as to be able to live with their conscience, and still practice a milder form of medicine relying more on hygiene.

As to immunization with vaccines this is another medical myth. Here is the evidence of the increase of Polio in States where Polio vaccination was compulsory.

1.- North Carolina, 78 cases in 1958 before compulsion, 313 cases in

1959 after compulsory shots.

2.- Connecticut, 45 cases in 1958 before compulsions, 123 cases in 1959

3.- Tennessee: 119 cases in 1958 before compulsion, 386 cases in 1959

4.- Ohio: 17 cases in 1958 before compulsory shots, 52 cases after

5.- Los Angeles, 89 cases in 1958 before, 190 cases in 1959 after the compulsory shots.

The Surgeon General Leonard Scheel overseeing the Polio eradication scheme said: "No batch of Vaccine can be proved safe before it is given to children" So they continue to promote vaccines that killed and paralyzed thousands. (Eleanor Bean) The supposed harmless Salk vaccine resulted in paralysis in the limb receiving the injection, which was diagnosed as something else. This is why oral vaccine was substituted for the Salk vaccine, because the digestive juices destroy the vaccine, or drugs like penicillin, when given by the mouth.

The 11th of May 1987, the Times of London published on its front page the News that the SMALL POX VACCINATION WAS SPREADING THE AIDS VIRUS. The essence of this affirmation is that the World Health Organization (WHO) in its 93rd campaign to eradicate small pox in the Third World (1967-1980) has set off an explosion of millions of cases of AIDS in

Africa, Brazil and Haiti. However the London Times news was hushed up completely in a blackout in the U.S.A., Reuters, U.P.I. etc. having no mention with smallest note even. It was evidently censored by the American Medical Association for fear that people would stop participation in vaccination schemes which is a major source of medical income.

The Science editor of the Times, Pierce Wright, listed the nations that have been vaccinated: Zaire 36 million, Zambia 18 million, Tarzania 15 million, etc. of which the diffusion of the SIDA virus coincides with the nations that were vaccinated. In Brazil the greatest campaign in South America to eradicate small pox has now the greatest incidence of SIDA in South America. With all the findings we only give only this brief note showing how the whole affair was treated in a censorship blackout in America.

We are living in the Age of Germ Warfare.

Disease is spread thru out the world by traitorous sabotage of those who pretend to be the guardians of our health. The very people they are said to serve are duped by these two faced medical authorities. Children are denied an education, adults intimidated against the knowledge of the truth and health, for the sake of medical profits.

Dr. Alexis Carrel in "Man Unknown" explained these immunization strategies thus: "The years of life which we have gained by the suppresion of acute diseases, diptheria, small pox, scarlet fever, typhoid fever, etc., are paid for by the long suffering and lingering deaths caused by chronic diseases, especially by cancer, diabetes, heart disease and stroke."

Rather than healing the body of its infected or diseased organs or parts, the medical doctors of the 20th century preferred to perform needless operations, removing the diseased part. One of the early expositions that Dr. Shelton made which was published by the New York Evening Graphic on Nov. 2nd 1928, commented upon by Doug Henning in his book, "Houdini, His Legend and Magic" which read as follows: "Herbert M. Shelton, Naturopath, in pointing out the ignorance of the medical and surgical practitioners, which has resulted in many deaths of public figures lately, declared today that nature provides for the protective gland when the appendix bursts and left alone the poison would be carried out of the system in the same manner all poisons are carried out".

William Howard Hay, M.D. in 1938 wrote: "Appendicitis is supposed to be an essentially surgical condition, and to hint that there is another possible aspect is to incur the lasting disrespect and wrath of any surgeon. Yet, in the practice of the writer (himself formerly sold out to the surgical idea in appendicitis), during the past 26 years there has not been one death from any form of this very common accident. No surgery was involved in any case even in 19 ruptured cases... Nothing was done except empty the colon as completely as possible and withhold everything digestive, even water, till the resulting abscess had matured and emptied again into its natural point of least resistance, the colon itself. When the rupture of the appendix occurs, there is at once formation of adhesive bands about the area, sequestering this completely, and it is unthinkable that nature can do this instantaneous job and then fail to maintain the barrier.

The surgeon opens the abdomen, breaks up this restraining wall of adhesions, and in doing so opens fresh lymph channels to further infection and 50% of his ruptured cases die, as he expects, but his ready alibi is always that the case was operated too late... In all over 400 cases of every type and degree of appendicitis have gone thru this simple process of emptying of the colon and correcting the diet, without any failure or one case that had to go thru the operative treatment". Dr. Shelton estimates that only 5% of the women operated for breast cancer actually have cancer.

Cancer is a dreaded killer among humans as well as beasts. Sir William Arthnot, British physician and surgeon stated: "There is one cause of disease and that is poison. We may take poison thru the air but we manufacture most of it within ourselves from the food we eat. In any case where I had the opportunity to verify it, I have found the patient suffering from chronic intestinal stasis and that the infection by cancer was the indirect consequence of the condition."

Another British physician, Ernest H. Tipper, M.R.C.S., attributed cancer to eating the wrong combinations of food. The combination of proteins and starches common among our people, such as bread with flesh foods is the cause of cancer which he specifically objects to, he claims. Dr. John Round, years ago in his thesis, "Flesh Eating and Cancer", claimed eagles and vultures, reptiles and other flesh eating animals frequently have cancer. Cancer in dogs, cats and other carnivorous domestic pets fed like humans have alarming rates of occurrence.

Yet cancer is rare in goats, sheep, horses, rabbits or unheard of. Cattle which are fed grains and many kinds of toxic substances instead of their natural food, have frequent cancer. Vegetarians get cancer eating eggs and milk occasionally. Interesting in this connection is the question of, "Why did Graham die early? The Hampshire Gazette Sept. 16, 1851 said, Dr. Sylvester Graham died at his residence in this town on Thursday morning last at the age of 57. He had been unwell for something like a year, suffering from rheumatism in his hands and lower limbs. A post mortem examination disclosed no diseases of the system which in the opinion of the medical examiners was sufficient to produce death, and the immediate cause of his decease, is thought to be, even contrary to the advice of his physician and friends, and the extreme exhaustion of the system, use of congress water a tepid bath. Dr. Alcott said that Sylvester Graham's father was 70 years older, inherited a feeble constitution, and Sylvester did not begin practice of his teaching till near forty, when his body was impaired by wrong habits. Our opinion is that Graham's rheumatism was like the gout that Benjamin Franklin complained about, that is caused by excessive use of grains, even the whole-grain Graham bread, as well as other seed foods such as nuts which he advocated. So after 40 years of abuse of bread, etc. with the reform of whole-grains, etc. they did not set well with him, and since in this time fruits and vegetables were not shipped fresh from the south in the winter, his death can well be attributed to the use of whole-grain bread, nuts and earth water which also contains calcareous acid forming substances. In the Dec. 30th 1891 Hampshire Gazette it adds "One of the habits of Dr. Graham was to bathe in Mill River every day, summer and winter. He cut a hole in the ice in winter, take off his clothes, stand on the ice in bare feet, take two dunkings and rub himself."

Another interesting aspect that Hygiene teaches is concerned with Intestinal Parasites given Dr. Shelton's Hygienic Review, May 1970. "Intestinal parasites do no trouble to those of normal digestive powers; those who have normal resistance. An intestinal tract that does not harbor decomposition and putrefaction will successfully resist an invasion of parasites and bacteria. Intestinal catarrh permits the inroads of parasites. So-called Amoebic dysentery is not caused by an amoeba, but by the factors of life that break down resistance, and provide a favorable habitat for the amoeba. Drugs to kill the amoeba add to the systemic impairment and do not restore the health of the patient. Patients with so-called amoebic dysentery suffer more from the treatment administered to them by specialists than they do from dysentery. Amoebic dysentery ends in recovery in two or three weeks if the patient is cared for properly and no amoebicides are given by mouth or enemas. These drugs cause inflammation, building ulcerative colitis and proctitis. The ulceration is then accredited to the parasites. Its is well known that parasites do not thrive in an empty colon and when deprived of a decomposing food supply upon which they live, they perish and the patient lives. This means that the surest and safest way to free the digestive tract of patients from it is to fast. This also aids in freeing the patient of his intestinal catarrh, after which digestion becomes normal. Thereafter a correct mode of living and sane eating will maintain a digestive tract in which parasites can find no lodgement. This plan of care works as effectively with tapeworm as with amoeba and hookworm.

Not only do Dr. Shelton and the Hygienists, as well as most drugless healers maintain that DRUGS DO NOT HEAL, but Kenneth Walker, M.A., M.D., F.R.C.S. says: "Thanks to the extraordinary recuperative powers of the human body and the resilience of the human mind, the patient generally managed thru-out the ages to recover health in spite of the vicissitude of treatment to which he has been subjected. Since 80 to 90% of patients will recover from their illness without any remedies at all, the great majority in those days recovered to the church's glory.

This fact of spontaneous cure explains the success of Christian Science, prayers by other church members, as well as harmless pills or treatments administered. The obvious fact is that prayers have less repressive effects upon the processes of life and give rise to no dangerous side effects. There is only 10 to 20% that can be accredited to being properly cared for, so faith healing is about the same as early hygienist's Orthopathy "let alone" or "do nothing" patient care of Doctors Jennings, Trall and Graham. Beside the British physician and surgeon we mentioned above, H.W. Haggard, M.D. says that "80% to 90% of all ailments get well of themselves under fair conditions, but most people imagine that such recoveries are positive cures."

"Our most violent poisons are our most potent medicines", said Martin Payne, M.D. L.L.D. "They act in the same way as the remote causes of disease. We do but cure one disease by producing another." (Institutes of Medicine, page 542) This is what the Hygienists have been preaching for over a century against medicine. Now even the medics recognize that Iatrogenic disease is more lethal than the original disease that physicians gave drugs for alleviating the patient's suffering.

With the maternity wards of hospitals taking over with facilities for surgery and the use of drugs there came a great lose of life at childbirth. As to the original female midwife being superior to the male midwife and hospital delivery, the use of anesthetics and physicians in 1719 Mrs. Elizabeth Phillips came to America from London, and when she died in 1761 at 76 in Charlestown, Mass. she had delivered three thousand births with no fatal accidents in her practice. In 1705 Mrs. Wait died in Dorchester, Mass. at 94 years of age when she had attended more than a thousand births without losing one. Mrs. Whitman of Marlboro, Vermont aged 87 had attended two thousand births without the loss of one patient.

Many physicians take their own lives when they discover drugs are killing their patients; some take up other occupations and many turn to the drugless professions to relieve their guilt. James F. Baldwin, M.D. F.A.C.S. the President of the Ohio State Medical Association said in his presidential address to the body already in 1920: "An exceedingly weak part of our position is such an enormous array of useless drugs as presented in our pharmacopoeia. No thinking observer can look over the pages of the book without being amazed at the credulity of a profession that tolerates such a farrago of nonsense, such a hodgepodge of trash."

Much of the faulty theories about drugs destroying diseases has been augmented by the belief that microorganisms or "germs" cause illness. Louis Pasteur is usually accredited with the origination of the idea that infectious diseases were caused by extremely small living organisms. However, in 1659, Kirchner, a Jesuit priest and mathematician with a crude microscope concluded that infectious diseases were caused by what he called little "living worms". Leuwenhoek with his improved microscope in 1675 was the first to actually observe and describe bacteria. Louis Pasteur was not a medical doctor, starting his studies with the fermentation of wine, beer and putrefaction. Studying diseases of the silkworm led to the study of germs, that a specific germ is absolutely responsible for the occurrence of a disease.

Hence, Pasteur developed his bacteriophobia, which his biographer Dr. Rene J. Dubos, describes as a fear of shaking hands, examining every bit of food he ate, the tableware, etc. for contaminating germs etc. As Dr. Dubos asserts, "The Germ Theory of fermentation and disease was based on the belief in the specificity and permanence of biological and chemical characteristics of microbial species". In other words, a specific microbe caused by a specific microbial species, which will always be remembered as Pasteur's Folly.

In brief, as Dr. Dubos wrote: "When nearly 60 years old, Pasteur discovered facts which were not in accord with his old concepts, (That disease germs were unchangeable in form and chemical properties)" Then he found that, "The presence in the body of a pathogenic agent is not synonymous with infectious disease". A certain germ may be present during a disease but this is not proof that such a germ was the cause of the disease. Pasteur was forced to acknowledge that germs are not the specific and preliminary cause, so he actually abandoned his theory of disease. We shall later show that a specific microorganism not only may change form and chemical properties with the change of toxins causing sickness beside germs not causing any kind of disease.

Before we return to describing Dr. Clements and Dr. Shelton's Orthopathy and Natural Hygiene reforms, in the first two or three decades of the 20th century, there was a tendency in slighting the important fundamentals and allowing allopathic medicine or surgery to adulterate the original Hygienic teachings. In the 1920-30s era, Bernarr Macfadden's "Physical Culture" magazine published advertisements about the Battecreek Sanitarium of John Harvey Kellogg, M.D., L.L.D., F.A.C.S. claimed to be the largest sanitarium in the world, and altho founded on Hygienic principles, gradually errors in needless surgery, and relaxed conformity got into the institution. Yet Battlecreek Sanitarium reigned in scientific training in nutrition, and the scientific world was hard put in keeping face, having to admit that flesh eating, alcoholism, smoking and dependence on drugs has caused the poor health, and high rate of delinquency beside mortality from incurable diseases. Dr. Kellogg provided trained dieticians to over 50 leading hospitals in the U.S.A., was the medical director and superintendent at the Battlecreek Sanitarium for 46 years and the editor of a monthly journal "Good Health" for 56 years. His book "The Natural Diet of Man" was a superb classic on the vegetarian diet. Dr. Kellogg's brother became even more known due to the breakfast cereals, such as corn flakes, all bran, etc. which were received in the sample parcels thru the mails addicting children to junk foods in the 1920-1930s.

Dr. Herbert Shelton's criteria on food was: "A FOOD IS A SUBSTANCE USABLE BY THE BODY AND IS TRANSFORMED INTO LIVE STRUC-TURE. A non-usable substance is a poison, and must be expelled. A drug is a poisonous substance that is of no use to the body, and worse, unites with living cells resulting in death in the cell."

This we have noticed in what the Hygienists defend as the only beverage that man should drink, the common well water, or water in streams and springs. In Latin America there are some dishonest people who sell milk with water added. So when the watered milk sours for its use as curds, the curds and whey both sink to the bottom of the container, since the lacto-bacterial culture is killed by the salt, limestone and iron oxide in common earth water that combines with the living cells. Thus, the body also rejects poisons that are often introduced by vomiting, diarrhea, and/or eruptions in the skin, and if unable to reject them, they destroy body cells.

Dr. Shelton's Hygienic Review was kind enough to print various advertisements for the author, Dr. Johnny Lovewisdom, but in the midst of them he published an article against "Pseudo-Hygiene" (June 1967) directed to a French language publication promoting the theories and practices of a man in South America "who is the polar opposite of a true Hygienist". So what is so objectionable with the French publication and the South American heretic to Shelton's Hygienic concepts? He says, "they have never hitherto been written in any books of so-called healing, nor taught in colleges nor recognized by healing professions... A genuine system of hygiene must be grounded on the principles of Nature. It cannot be based on Metaphysics and mysticism".

First, considering that the quarrel is on religious grounds, as a Christian it certainly has a backing in many colleges and universities. As a Buddhist, I believe I am qualified to say Dr. Shelton and the Western World does not realize that the Buddha based his teaching and beliefs on experience. Thus he did not consider the unproved theories about Brahman or God as practical in his way of life. As to living on live or raw foods such as herbs, vegetables and fruits and curds which we and the earliest representations of the Buddha seem to imply, this we found most practical. In Ecuador only coconuts are abundant in the coast, elsewhere only weevil ridden nuts from U.S.A. are available. Some Hygienists allow curds, cottage cheese and other such products, as Shelton does in this transition diet, so this is what experience will prove as the most reliable protein to be used with salads and fruits live food diets.

The French publication supporting the South American was probably by Dr. A. Mosseri of Rigney Nonneuse, France, or Dr. Jauvais of Bordeaux, France. Now Dr. Shelton holds that the South American's teaching is the "polar opposite" of Hygiene, and the French publication teaching Hygiene as Orthobionomics, are clues as to the subtle implication against Hygienists teachings being unfounded on Bible-Christian theology. There had been differences between Jennings, Graham and Trall, as well as with early Hygienists and the recent modern ones, but none had been so captivated by the unsound theories and terminology as Dr. Shelton's school, so as to oppose all religious references. Thus, not only did Shelton oppose what he named "Pseudo-Hygiene", but also published articles on "Body and Spirit", "Churchianity and Medicine", "Theresa Neumann is Dead", etc. separating Shelton's Hygiene from most all of its early pioneers who based their teachings on Spirit as the Source of Life, God and the Bible.

The mention of Theresa Neumann specially pointed your writer out since he wrote considerably about her and others who did not eat among the Church, Saints and Eastern Yogis. This even influenced Dr. George R. Clements who had been the early publisher of the "How To Live" journal and courses on Orthopathy, to withdraw, having turned to Breatharianism, under pseudonyms of Kenyon Klamonti and Prof. Hilton Hotema, noticing Shelton's frustration. The Hygienic Review thus continued with the slogan, "Let us have Truth Though the Heavens Fall" and the statement combined with "How To Live". Clements had based his books and "How to Live" articles on Bible quotations, in the same Hygienist tradition.

Now Dr. Clements and Dr. Goldwasser taught Devolution, and Orthopathy first taught by Dr. Jennings was based on Vitalism, the self healing power of the body which likewise is of Divine origin, rather than being founded on evolution. "Vitalism" is defined by Webster's as "The doctrine that life is, in part, self-determining and self-evolving; opposed to mechanism". Charles Darwin (1809-1882) came after the early Hygienists, with his theory of "Evolution" which holds "that all species of plants and animals developed from earlier forms by hereditary transmission of slight variations in successive generations, those forms surviving which are best adapted to the environment, by natural selection and survival of the fittest."

"Bionomics" is defined by Webster's as ecology; "the branch of biology that deals with adaptations of living things to their environment". So, Ortho-bionomics according to Shelton is "the correct management of life", or a synonym for Natural Hygiene. Yet, correct adaptations to environment are a biology which is based on Darwin's theory. Hence, as we shall see, that the Biological Sciences are a headless horseman. Evolution in biology refers to the development of a species, organism or organ from its original or rudimentary state to its present completed state, phytogeny or ontogeny; (b) the obsolete theory that a germ cell contains the fully developed traits in a miniature form; theory of preformation; (c) the theory now generally accepted, that all species of plants and animals developed from earlier forms by hereditary transmission of slight variations in successive generations. These theories do not account for the direction and guiding forces that gave the Creation of the earth and the heavens. Shelton's "Truth though the heavens fall" was thus smothered by the "testimony of Truth given John" who said, "man cannot receive anything unless it be given... He that comes from heaven is abode all." (Jn.1:8;3:27, 31)

The theory that the whole universe was evolved with a "big bang" haphazardly without intelligent order or laws puts the end product or intelligent man and gods out of the scene, proving its impossibility from the start. With God all things became possible.

The Self-Healing Life-process that Jennings attributed to living organisms in his Orthopathy was based on the definition of Vitalism, and thus was really the "polar opposite" to Darwin's theory of Evolution and the Biological Sciences that include Ortho-bionomics that flourished after Jennings, Graham and Trall and their followers. Dr. Jennings "Theory of Human Life" quoted John as to the "Word of Life", which is the "Fiat" of the Almighty Creator who created the heavens and earth in Genesis. "In the beginning was the Word, and the Word was with God, and the Word was God... All things were made by Him." The Fiat was the Wisdom, identified biblically as the Word of Life, that made it all, without exotic theories of chemical and physical formations evolving into higher intelligences from nothing in a godless world. A Higher Spiritual Intelligence or Divine Wisdom guided Life in all its forms into an intelligent order and natural laws of being. Intelligent order and natural laws of an Omniscient Power were not the product of chaos.

Likewise, Dr. Russell Trall based his Hygieo-Therapeutic College and claims of the Hygienic System and School, on the vitalistic doctrine. His treatise presented to the New York Senate gaining outstanding approval for the College rested on "strict obedience to every one of the laws which the Creator has implanted in the vital domain of that being which He has fearfully and wonderfully formed and fashioned in his own image, make to rank in the scale of being a "little lower than the angels", and endowed with eternal and god-like attributes. He explains the theory of Vitality, the life force or vital powers, and reaffirms Dr. Jennings idea of the self-healing power of the body due to the vital principle without external medication. Due to Jennings' exposition in Orthopathy, and the great success among Hygienic practitioners for over a quarter century, he received top honors in his time.

In turn, while the graduated medical doctors Jennings and Trall are ignored by Webster's dictionary, it recognizes "Sylvester Graham, (1794-1851) as American physician, designating or made of unsifted whole wheat flour, as graham crackers". Accrediting him as a physician was due, or should have been due to his introduction of fresh fruits and vegetables into the nation's diet, beside fresh air, bathing and other hygienic principles into the healing of cholera and other ailments in hundreds of victims without any loss of patients, while ordinary drug treatment lost most of their clients.

Thus the Vitalogical Sciences were established on the Life Principle, so that Vitalogical Healing is Healing with Life, as we wrote in our course on "Vitalogical Healing and Hygiene" in 1968. At the time (1968) your author had made very little research into the early hygienists, Jennings, Graham and Trall, having read only Dr. Shelton's Hygienic Review, which lacks biblic mention, so independently he began teaching with reference continually to the bible Scripture, as the early hygienists had done. For instance, Dr. Shelton affirms "there is no live water", which your author refers to as a basic principle in diet, as "living water", ignoring the fountainhead of Hygiene in the Gospel. The living water that Jesus gave or prescribed is the basis of his teaching of baptism and rebirth or regeneration for: "The (living) water I shall give him shall become in him a fountain of life springing up into Life Everlasting". (Jn.4:14)

We wondered as to how we might rescue Orthopathy and Natural Hygiene from animalism. "Animalism", Webster defines as (1) Animal qualities; (2) the doctrine that men are mere animals with no soul or spiritual qualities. This seemed to be Shelton's aberration in fixations, since he could not bear to have people relate to him about God or Karma-free living, due to his recent past in moral standards. The true Hygienist, whom Shelton classifies as frugivorous, are only the anthropoid primates. Yet the mighty gorilla, which he lauds in "Health for the Millions" said to chew his food with 32 teeth like man, considers wild celery as his favorite food and weighs 500 lbs. is not a fruitarian. Encyclopedia Brittanica says no more than 15% of the gorilla diet is fruit, usually much less, so over 85% is wild greens, plants or shoots. In that case man is essentially herbivorous. But since the other anthropoids, baboon, chimpanzee, orangutan, etc. are on average half fruit and other half greens eaters, this may compare correctly with an ideal frugivore. However, to classify man with merely non-spiritual animals, or animalistic, departs from the man Dr. Jennings taught to be created by the Fiat or Word of the Creator thru the vital principle, and which Dr. Trall said was given laws by the Creator, and fashioned in His own Image and likeness, fearfully and wonderfully made, endowed with eternal and god-like attributes. As Dr. Goldwasser said, "Man from the Spirit, lo and behold, Is man of a deeper and higher mold..."

However, what most obviously characterizes the 20th century teachers of Hygiene and Orthopathy was the effeminate hairless faces, women-like dandies, which include Tilden, Shelton, Clements, Goldwasser and their followers. In this they desert the Nazarene Jesus in ancient Nazarite-Essene vows, even if they touch not the corpse of dead or use no alcoholic beverages. Natural Living and Hygiene needs to be consistent thru-out its practice, and not taking what is easy and popular, and shunning what is not convenient. The hair is a living part of the body, and when the hair is cut it bleeds wasting valuable elements that could be deprived from the brain, nerves, hearing, sight, endocrine glands, etc. In the case of fingernails and toenails, modern man wearing shoes and using fingers in typing and other work which may cause ingrown toenails, cracking, etc. there is a legitimate precaution, but cutting hair removes dignity of the Creator's image of god-like man.

There is also the case of a Chiropractor who lived a short while in Loja, and when he and his wife had business to do in other cites, they would leave their four children with us, knowing we only ate raw salads and fruits. So we had them do a "workshop" fixing their own food, but they were negligent, using large grater on carrots that should be grated fine, leaving cabbage leaves in chunks rather than finely sliced, etc. so when they evacuated into our compost-outhouse the salad came out undigested and unassimilated. However they did make use of the vegetable juices and tree-ripe fruits. Occasionally, some uninformed neighbor would give them cooked rice, etc. but when their father found out he would wallop their bottom side. When they moved to Quito, he and his wife would eat away from home, and soon it was known that occasionally they had a hamburger and other cooked foods on such occasions. So, finally they tried to get back gradually going to a vegetarian restaurant where they served cooked meals. However the owners had gotten word of the happenings, and that in order to be served, they must bring their whole family, so the children would benefit from example rather than from fear of a spanking. They thus let their children eat what they ate, and going back to Texas, after the Chiropractor earned enough to retire, thus the children all joined the marines, still in the father's guidance for discipline in their lives.

However, we do not pretend to be the polar opposite of Dr. Shelton's Hygienic System, but rather count ourselves benefactors. To make reparations for points wherein he strayed from the ideal, he made himself a hard task-master. For instance there was not to be any grating of carrots, no juicing of vegetables, fine slicing of lettuce, cabbage and other leaves, which should be served whole as they come from the garden, without oxidation that destroys many valuable life elements. He did however make exception for the edentulous members of our race, who lack the 32 teeth and 200 lbs. pressure to masticate food like the gorilla. The point is well founded, but in practice one has to either make the effort to chew food, or alternately develop the effort of juicing, grating, etc. along with a rapid way to ingest the food before there is much oxidation. In the author's first course on diet, "Spiritualizing Dietetics, Vitarianism", many good points were made, but eventually it condemned even the use of vegetables, leaving only juicy fruits for food, and then hoped to give up even fruit eating to live a Heavenly Life without Eating. Needless to say, I was not gifted with such powers even if some rare instances have appeared of people doing such things. However in each extreme that I have tried to comply with or challenge our students have been warned of the limits of what is practical, beneficial and what pitfalls in error are to be avoided.

In the case of dairy products and cooked foods, my judgement in avoiding dairy products for 30 years turned out to be an obstacle in a strictly live or raw food diet. The raw food enzymes in bacterially cultured milk enabled the digestion of a vast variety of vegetable foods with all the necessary food elements, while the cooking of food not only destroyed many food elements but did not make healthful adaptations in palatability and digestion in comparable improvement. Yet, while clabber, or curds with the whey as a whole food, answered the need for salad dressings, in time we found that even tho the whey did contain calcium and other minerals, it was the cause of blood acidity since lactic acid is the waste product of muscular activity. In the final analysis, the curds or cottage cheese was the preferable adaptation even if it was not a whole food, unless we consider it as removing a waste product as when one does cutting off pineapple, hard avocado, or other inedible fruit skins. In practice, Dr. Shelton, Dr. Esser, and other modern Natural Hygienists include cottage cheese in their menus, at least in transition if not permanently.

The greatest challenges for man which one in a million not only include life without eating, but also life approaching everlasting. In "Spiritualizing Dietetics, Vitarianism" we quoted William L. Lawrence's article in "Look" (3/24/53),- "You May Live Forever" who reported on Dr. Oscar Schott's findings that there exists in every living creature, be it a tapeworm or a human being, the seed of immortality, a seed of the phoenix as it were, entirely different and apart from the egg and sperm cells that give rise to offspring, the normal perpetuation of the species. Verily, the fountain of youth sought thru the ages, has been identified by Dr. Schott as the regenerative scar tissue that keeps the body in constant repair thru-out life, and without which life would be much shorter than it actually is. It is these very phoenix cells molded by the Sculptor of life that rebuild every cell and organ, with the exception of the brain, and the central nervous system about every 7 years. When man has at last succeeded in definitely isolating the Sculptor and in determining the sort of tools and the working conditions it requires, the goal scientists universally will be reached in the not too distant future, man will have learned the secret of immortality".

Well, lo and behold, it can be told that the Doctor of Orthopathy Jacob Goldwasser, with the information given by William H. Goodell, wrote a book which was named "The Truth Will Smash Civilization" which was too unbelievable to become popular. They told of Master Jain Bio-chemists at Mount Abu in India, who had hair trailing down to the earth behind them, one of which is 750 years old, photographed in a local newspaper as documentary evidence, with companions whose ages exceed over the patriarchs of the Bible even reaching 1,400 years. They ate only figs, a handful a day, rarely olives, wore only a rope fiber loin cloth, and slept in caves. (See our book "Those Strong, Powerful and Extraordinary Vegetarians" for greater detail) The western scientist wants tools to play with in laboratories, and will never face nor isolate the Sculptor of Life. Otherwise, he would go sit at the feet of these Masters who today, as always, know how to live forever.

PART TWO: VITALOGICAL HYGIENE

THE ESSENE GENESIS OF THE PRISTINE ORDER OF PARADISIAN PERFECTION

THE INITIAL PARADISIAN CONSECRATION

John declared, "In the beginning was the Word, and the Word was with God; and the Word was God." Just what was the Word which he referred to? The Word was "Beresith", in Hebrew being the first Word with which the Book of Generations of our Holy Scripture begins with, also known best as Genesis, meaning thus "In the beginning", or to proclaim the History of Creation. The next word is "Elohim", so designated because Elohim is the God who created all that was created, and since "In the beginning God created heaven and earth", the first testimony spoken by Elohim in the plural. Thus, John considered the Word as Wisdom in God's Creation, as also was the meaning before the fallacious theory of evolution and modifications elaborated by atheistic sciences.

Then, before anything else on earth, the Elohim created by their Word, or Wisdom, and brought forth on earth, "every green herb, and such as yieldeth seed according to its kind, and the tree that beareth fruit, having seed each one according to its kind. And the Elohim saw that it was good." Herein is the precept that herbs and fruits contain a reproductive substance that they give forth for growing their own kind.

Then "the Elohim created man in their own image, in the likeness of the Elohim they created him: Male and female they created them." Being the likeness of Gods; the Sons of God were God, and God the Creator was the Father which John referred to, the Son being the Word by which all was made. In actual translation it was not possible to keep the gender correct, since God's image is both male and female, two, and thus the first man was two in gender, male and female like the Creator. Consequently, the Word, the Son of God was androgynous (and not what produces male offspring only, or androgenous) being male and female, and unlike other creatures described in this first chapter. Furthermore, the androgynous Son was created with distinct attributes to "Increase and multiply, and fill the earth", with herbs, fruit trees, creatures and what God exemplified in the Word of Wisdom. "The Son cannot do anything of himself, but what he seeth the Father doing, for what things soever he doth, these the Son also doth in like manner." (Jn.5:19) This should explain why the Sons of God are born androgynous, without bestial reproduction, immaculately begotten by the Word thru Virgin Birth, or as John states: "Unless a man be born again of living water and the Holy Spirit, he cannot enter the Realm of God."

71

The Sons of God, whom John thus qualifies saying, "Committeth not sin, for the seed abideth within him..." in perpetual continence enabled by perpetually partaking of the Holy Communion for the Holy Table, or Altar, of God's Creation with the Word. "Behold, I have given every herb bearing seed upon the earth, and all trees that bear fruit which yield seed after their own kind, to you for food... And God saw all things that he had made, and they were very good."

In Spanish, the word for blessing is "bendecir", rooting from bien decir meaning to say or declare good, as these Divine Words declare as to man's food being fruit and green herbs. It is defined as "alabar" or praise, glorify or celebrate. (2) It also means to consecrate. However, the English word "blame" is derived from "bledsian" the Anglo-Saxon root is blood, sprinkling with blood, and thus according to Webster's of evil omen for us. The word "Consecrate" is not derived directly from such roots, being defined as (1) to set apart as holy, make or declare sacred, dedicate or devote. So in relation to our reference to man's God-Given food "consecrate" is most appropriate. The Spanish equivalent is "Consagrar" meaning to make sacred, roots auspiciously in "make holy".

Men have pretended to make altars holy and blessed with human and animal blood, bread and wine, but the Holy Writ begins by God consecrating fruits and green herbs (or vegetables) as the truly good and only holy food for man. The first chapter of Isaiah likewise condemns such bloody sacrifices, incense and festivals of drunkenness and harlotry: "To what purpose do you offer me the multitude of your victims, sayeth the Lord? I am full, I desire not holocausts of rams and fattlings and blood of calves and lambs and buck-goats." Furthermore, in chapter 3:7 the Lord says, "I am no healer and in my house there is no bread or clothing", condemning the altar loaves of show-bread and the elaborate vestments of priests who offer such vain sacrifices. Only man, the sinner, for whom the earth was cursed (Gen.3:17), eats bread thereof in the sweat of his face, and drinks wine yielding intoxication disgracing himself like Noah, and falsely claims God said all this is good and holy. God offers no wholesomeness or health therein, refusing to be our healer as long as we partake of bread, wine, flesh and blood.

The active members of the HEAVENLY ECCLESIA OF THE LIVING GOD IN AEONIAN REVIVIFICATION, and of the PRISTINE ORDER OF PARADISIAN PERFECTION celebrate the true Holy Eucharist, whenever they eat; moreover they do not desecrate God-Given Food, fruits and green herbs, by saying Grace before meals, or substituting Sacraments invented by men, and much less by cooking or processing these foods. What God made very good in the beginning, is holy, sacred and consecrated as the Tree of Life Everlasting, and by joyful acceptance we acknowledge our thanks for what God alone consecrated. Good will in God's Will is our thanks, "grateful acknowledgment of something received by or done for one", according to Webster's.

Ceremony, ritualism and sacramental sacrifices, like vicarious atonement are a gruesome, ghastly stigmata that have frightened our gently humanity away from the Christian Religion in its association with ancient Hebrew history, and only John's Gnosticism unveils the Pristine Order of Paradisian Perfection in the first book and first chapter by which mankind may be rescued to embrace an Everlasting Essene Religion in a truly scientific philosophy from the crass abandon in materialistic atheism.

No longer will men drench their robes in the blood of beasts, nor feign imitation by a so-called bloodless sacrifice, yet celebrated for a bloody victim in mock glorification, supposedly receiving life because a man died on a cross giving us his life to save us, a gory tradition of superstition. With a peaceful heart, Paradisians will again aggregate in body, or at least soul, to partake in the God-Given Sacred Repast in innocence in initial silent invocation allowing the Creator to consecrate our life sustenance.

In poignant reminiscence again we cite from the Essene Book of Adam of Eve: "Seth the elder, tall and food, with a fine soul, and a strong mind, stood at the head of his people, and tended to them in innocence, penitence and meekness, and did not allow one of them to go down to Cain's children. Because of their own purity they were named the sons of God, and they were with God. Seth and his children did not like earthly works, but gave themselves to heavenly things. Seth and his children dwelt on the mountain below the Garden; they sowed not, neither did they reap; they wrought no food for the body, not even wheat; but only offerings. They ate of the fruit and of the trees well flavored that grew on the mountain where they dwelt. Seth often fasted forty days as did also his eldest children. For the family of Seth smelled the smell of the trees in the Garden, when the wind blew that way. They were happy, innocent, without sudden fear, there was no jealousy, no evil action, no hatred among them. There was no animal passion; from their mouth among them went forth neither foul words nor curse; neither evil counsel nor fraud."

Only with the incipience of our modern Pristine Order of Paradisian Perfection did we realize that these long lost Scriptures contained verifiable facts capable of confirmation. As a Paradisian Elder in 1974, well beyond the mid-century period, this Patriarch was upliftingly complemented when a young sister in the Paradisian Paradigm massaging his feet, described how delightfully fragrant the soles smelled, like the fruit or blossoms of pineapple, papayas, and oranges. Undeniably such a witness of the aroma exuding from someone, whose mid-day meal consists of these very fruits, shows that the author of the "Book of Adam and Eve" spoke of people who were really living in the Paradisian Example, and not some fictitious imagination or ideals of dreamers. All of us know the repulsive smell when a carnivorous or granivorous person takes off their shoes to remove sweat-filed socks, or even a vegetarian who uses a can of baked beans to dress their salad, and the resultant stench like "all-get-out"! Likewise, their bodily perspiration is so fetid as to compare only with menstrual blood or seminal loss decomposition.

Moreover, even in our tiny group we noticed the change of the color of the iris of the eyes, from brown to blue, as well as the bleaching of chestnut color hair turning into blond, as well as black to brown. After Dr. Bernard Jensen of Escondido, California visited us, we received his masterpiece on Iridiagnosis, in which he tells of similar phenomena among people living on raw uncooked food.

The healing of menstrual bleeding and wasteful seminal losses is the crowning achievement in occurrences while living on organically grown fresh fruits and vegetables with least of avocados, bananas, dates, or other highly concentrated sources of calories. We shall omit repeating other rarefications in body vibrancy in substance, so as to overcome gravity, giving physical levitation, an extension of the present body into multiple etheric duplicate forms, the super-conscious Samadhi traces, clairvoyance, telepathy and other "gifts" experienced thru the practice of Vitalogical Hygiene, other than this mention now herewithin, it does show that when I named my first book on this subject, "Spiritualizing Dietetics,-Vitarianism", the meaning was the opposite to what is meant by "materialization" of people's bodies, - which was a point that the Omangod Press editors never grasped, by shortening our title to "Spiritual Diet, Vitarianism". With these sensually perceptible phenomena, in the aura and the etheric vibrations of emanations seen by spiritually developed persons, there is the astonishingly brilliant colors either in blue or golden tints, just as living "or raw" foods such as fresh fruits and vegetables radiate similar radiant energies under the microscope, in contrast to the opaque, inert and dense vibration of dead cooked foods. As to storing Prana into dynamic potentials by the practice of breathing exercises of Eastern Yoga, that has met with an overwhelming challenge from our Western Vitalogical Hygiene which is able to surpass such artificial routes of purification.

Altho only a few of the authors of the books of the Old Testament were true Essenes, and likewise among the New Testament writers some were Gnostic Apostles trained by John, the Essene, there is fully enough material to be found on our Vitalogical Sciences for a material, mental and spiritual apprehensive grasp, enabling their practice in daily life among those open to the Divine Receptive Will of the Spirit of the Paradisian New Age. Of particular favorable coordination and good omen in the priesthood of the laity, is the full participation of women. Most often it is the fair sex that prepares and serves for participation at the Paradisian Eucharistic Table of the "Body and Blood of the Spiritual Jesus, which John so vividly describes in his Gospel, otherwise known as the Living Water of the juices, and the Living Bread meaning Food or "flesh" of fruits and vegetables. Empty purposes would only await women obtaining equality with male priests in the antiquated system of ceremony, ritual and sacramental sacrifices, rooted in ancient superstitions as to the vicarious redemption received from a gory victim, or the substitution of bread and wine in place of a human victim-symbolic consolation, food and drink of sinners cast out of the Garden of Eden.

What God consecrated as "very good" and holy needs not man's nor woman's artifice in hypocritical sham ceremony and invocations. Usually, it was not just men of the priestcraft, but likewise women who cooked and served the meals of those who were the faithful Christians, or other religions, who in reality desecrated fruits and vegetables from their natural goodness to please mankind in general. So what will be worthy in the Paradisian New Age, now, is fresh organic fruits and vegetables served clean but naturally wholesome. The failure of the monetary economic system netting complete inflation will make men and women both home-makers and providers, consecrated as Co-Creators of Paradise.

Furthermore, let us have altars dedicated to Life for the birds, the bees, the squirrels, and various animals, who also hunger and thirst like man for the fruits and vegetables of our gardens. This best achieved with compost piles located around or surrounding the garden, where the skins, excess seeds, spoiled and defective fruits and vegetables are deposited, where a fresh layer contains the delicacies which the various animal friends covet. They will be so busily at work that they will never notice the garden produce growing among the bushes, tree and plant leaves, vines, etc. hidden, immature, and not suited usually for their immediate consumption.

This also answers as an alternative to what many farmers suggest as "cures" against garden predators in using poisons, dead predators to warn others, and other means claimed effective, but in good reason may rebound on such incompassionate ones as altars of death. Jesus of the Gospels exemplified our paradigm by throwing out the doves, the lambs, and other livestock sold as clean sacrificial victims, beside the money-changers who are the real dealers of this fallacious system depicted as of the Lord. Yahweh, substituted usually with title "Lord" was the tribal God of the Hebrews, whose Scriptures declare Yahweh was pleased by animal fat and victims sacrificed to it, altho dead carcasses require burial to avoid the decomposing stench and air pollution. If one will examine parts cut away from fruits, vegetable parts, etc., one will find enough or plenty of good food, more effectively removed by animal claws, beaks, teeth etc. than human eating utensils. Let us have Altars for Life as the Elohim preached as the Word of Wisdom.

Free from the hoaxes of superstitions invented by Science, we are yet going to find: "Man from the Spirit, lo and behold, is man of a deeper and higher mold." The Elohim recorded God's creation of the human species in our Holy Scriptures in their first chapter, while Darwin doubted that Evolution was viable even in theory.

PART TWO: VITALOGICAL HYGIENE, HEALING AND RELATED NATURAL VITALOGICAL SCIENCES

When your author completed his first book on diet, "SPIRITUALIZING DIETETICS,-VITARIANISM" in 1954, the objectives were ethical, esthetical, moralistic and purposefully for the spiritual upliftment of mankind. Altho the Vitalogical Sciences deal ecologically with all aspects of human life and man's environment, yet the way in life that men live depends basically upon the most neglected aspect, systems of feeding.

Vitarianism basically involved the God-Given Design of feeding upon fruits and vegetables as living foods, with the exclusion of seeds and positively all flesh foods of animal origin. The exclusion of seeds, the reproductive parts and substance of plants is the most radical departure from common dietary practices of man, and thus it is emphasized more because generally today abstinence from flesh foods (fish, fowl included as flesh) is nearly universally accepted as healthful, and is frequently prescribed by physicians.

The chief argument against plant seminal substance is because it contains, contrary to purposefulness in feeding, reproductive enzymes which subtract and divide from the integrity of the human constitution, rather than add or multiply the benefits of nutrition, which is the objective of eating, sleeping, and other human proclivities.

Enzymes are defined as any of various organic substances that are produced in plant and animal cells and cause changes in other substances by catalytic action. One of the most authoritative writers on enzymes, Dr. Edward Howell, in his book "Enzyme Nutrition" confirms the author's findings as to the adversity of seeds in human nutrition. Only living foods contain enzymes, and thus coincide with the Vitalistic powers of fresh uncooked fruits and vegetables, confirming the purpose of Vitalogical Hygiene and Healing based on Vitalism rather than mere chemical and physical properties. Altho coincident with, but independent from findings of your present author, Dr. Edward Howell affirms that plants do have enzyme-inhibitors, or "anti enzymes" contrary to the purpose of food and human metabolism. When vegetables are stored too long, they develop a bitter taste, lose their succulent properties, emphatically seen in carrots, potatoes, etc. when left in the ground from one season to the next. Seeds have completed the seed-forming process, and like the seminal substance of animals and humans, contain the same reproductive enzymes, if applied to nutrition. Thus, raw seeds of plants cause seminal losses and menstruation in humans. Seeds contain anti-enzymes and thus they oppose or inhibit normal nutrition, and metabolism, in vitalistic properties. However, when they are cooked like other foods, they lose their enzymes, and become an unbalanced and pathological burden in relation to nutrition. They no longer catalyze the assimilation of the many amino acids, minerals and other factors necessary for complete health, and produce the enfeebled and repeatedly ailing organisms common to civilized mankind of our world today.

On this point of enzymology, we make our first distinction now in Vitalogical Hygiene and Healing in relation to Natural Hygiene, or "Orthobionomics" taught by the late Dr. Herbert M. Shelton, since he admits, "It is customary to include nuts in the category of fruits, altho it is the seed, rather than the seed carrying organ that we eat." Rodents such as rats and squirrels are not frugivorous, nor fruitarians, altho they both eat fruits and nuts. Vegetable greens, avocados, etc. contain all the necessary amino acids if eaten with large "wash basin" sized bowls of salad, rather than a mere supplementary relish for concentrated proteins as customary today. Altho Dr. Shelton and his modern Hygienists do not forbid cottage cheese or curds, included in their diets, yet many Hygienists are strictly against any animal products. As a Vegan for 30 years myself, refusing any animal products for food, to survive in modern world conditions, curds from milk were found necessary, due to the destruction of the body's own enzyme synthesizing functions especially in the intestines due to pesticides used on foods besides the voluntary or involuntary use of drugs. Thus, one must open one's mind to the facts in the present situation, that milk from cows, goats, mares, buffalo, etc. were intended by nature as food for something, altho only in the infant stage. Thus, it becomes necessary to mature, or ripen, milk into curds, which are bacterial plants grown in milk for mature human nutrition. Also, fresh cow's milk lacks the enzymes necessary for its digestion, altho some people are able to synthesize the necessary enzymes within their bodies.

Likewise, many fruits cannot be eaten when picked, avocados need to ripen soft, bananas need to ripen after picking them hard or green for flavor, apples of many types must mellow in flavor, as do pears, all of which are the work of enzymes in the ripening process, similar to the ripening of curds in milk in producing food for mature humans. While we were pioneering a new location at Shambhala Sanctuary and I still lived in Vilcabamba in 1980, my companion used to bring me a week's supply of fruits and milk uncontaminated with modern chemical toxins from the new region with a donkey. After a few hours bouncing up and down in boxes atop the donkey, the milk had fragrant fresh butter collected on top of the buttermilk, and the papayas, ripe bananas, pineapple, and other fruit that was ripe was of a delicious flavor like divine nectar almost unimaginable, due to the enzymatic action. Also if apples are still green, bananas and other fruit are still green, such green fruit has a great amount of enzyme inhibitors, and even if you put them in a drawer, plastic bag or container enclosed well, they may still fail to ripen faster. No, you need some ripe fruit to be enclosed with the green fruit for enzymatic action ripening the fruit instead of inhibiting it.

Next, as to the frequent moral problems of making cows, goats or other animals our nurse-maids, etc. since at this stage they lack full validity. Animal life in milk-giving animals would cease if they were all butchered or otherwise eliminated ecologically. Moreover, by providing pastures and protection from environmental traffic, poisoning, etc. there is a symbiotic relationship, since cows or other milk animals cannot build their own "cow meadows" in long gone wilderness areas, and in turn, man receives sustenance for his kind thru the tender loving care of milk providing companions in symbiosis. This Paradisian relationship was best illustrated in our translation of "La Montana Azul", quoted in our own treatise "Maha Maitreyana Mandala-Shambhala-1981.

"After writing her esoteric text on the "Secret Doctrine", Mdme. Helen P. Blavatsky went to relax and write freely in Russian, her native tongue, telling of the "Land of the Blue Mountain", in a beautiful and factual description of these mountains, 40 miles inland from Malabar on the west coast of India. There, existing in a comparatively modern world, she found such an antediluvian tribe like the "children of Seth" which we describe, and which she likened to the family of Enoch. The Sanskrit name for the Blue Mountains is composed of "Nilam" or blue, and "Guiri", mountains, that is, "Nilguiri" of which this surviving exemplary tribe, the Toddes, consisting of 700 men, is a part of numerous later arrivals, who also have a contrasting nature like the children of Cain and Abel to the Sethians. Virtually being a White Brotherhood, and practicing White Magic, as Mdme. Blavatsky describes their spiritual characteristics, also it uncovers many stories of giants like the biblical antediluvians, on their Mount of Sepulchres, one of the graves being reported a half dozen times the size of the their modern survivors, who even today are still very tall, no one of the Toddes being less than six foot three inches tall, and who say their forefathers were twice as tall as they are. In turn, at that same mountain, the "Black Magicians" practicing hypnotism to get what they need, live as hunters, being flesh eaters of the jungles, are 3 foot dwarfs, none of which seldom ever challenges the Toddes. Like in the Gnostic and Essene Scriptures of their forefathers, these Toddes never eat flesh or kill anything, neither do they possess or make weapons, not even a knife.

They neither sow nor reap, their chil dren remain always in naked innocence, but their adults were clothed in white raiment that resemble a
toga. We read of the Essenes, Therapeuts and Christian hermits or monks
attempting to live chaste lives, eating baked bread, salt and water alone,
rarely vegetables, and we readily see why they had to live segregated
in male groups, not trusting the moody, changeable nature of women
influenced by the moon and menstrual cycles, taking refuge in burning
obstinacy, feeling sure as the sun, of militant males. In turn, the fluidic
natural goodness of these children of the forest followed the ripening of
juicy fruits of the Blue Mountains, as if the giant boa constrictors, fierce
tigers and other dangerous beasts never existed at ones every step, which
for so long made the region inaccessible.

One of the protectors, with whom the Toddes shared a Symbiotic existence for survival was the giant breed of buffalo that they alone possessed. What ordinary people understand as their God and wisdom,
colored by self-praise, the Toddes attribute to their buffalo: rather than
wisdom or God being their intuitive influence, they would repeat, "the
buffalo told us so". Missionaries spent years nearby preaching Christianity to them, and in the end they were answered with, "What need do we
have for your gods if we have our buffalo!" Observing the diet, the way
of life and behavior of the outside world, they had good reason to avoid
all civilized people. There was never a lie told by them, they never cov-
eted and much less stole anything, never harmed or killed anything, yet
they had no word for God, cross, prayer, religion, sin etc. since they had
no need for them. Mankind has substituted words for what people lack
in goodness, love, truth, etc. from an intangible spiritual source of inner
feeling and knowing.

The Blue Mountains have a flora consisting of delicious fruits of lands
and climates, much like our equatorial Andes. There are pineapple,
bananas, and other tropical fruits lower down, and higher up apples,
raspberries and all kinds of temperate fruits and berries, being only 11
degrees north of the equator, which the Toddes ate and scattered the seed
of everywhere, along with lotuses, palms, etc. as well as pine and birch.
However, unlike the modern fruitarians with poor teeth from their childhood diets and unbalanced market fruits being poisoned with toxic substances that destroy metabolism, and unbalanced by farming methods,
the Toddes had beautiful, sound, white teeth even in old age. Their eyes
were blue, gray or hazel, reflecting the purity of body, which with white
racial origins equal to Caucasians in skin color, matched their Nordic tall
stature, bespeaking Hyperborean antiquity. Their buffalo, adorned with
musical bells, with whom they commune visibly at milking time much
like a ritual, share their mysteries, at their forest sanctuaries, are the

solemn witness as to why they are such a solitary tribe of sanctity, bearing beautiful bodies as well as souls. They will not use food given to them, nor even the milk of other buffalo, knowing the sacred goodness of their own unpolluted forest. Altho our source did not indicate it directly, but since they were able to serve curds to rarely encountered explorers, it testifies that in their vats of milk storage, they made a bacterial culture, or clabber, as do many long-lived people, altho the Toddes did this with detained dedication and blessing of this as a sacred food. Only the celibate elders were allowed to milk or touch their buffalo, those who had children being classified as mortals among them, just as milk is a pre-puberty food for mammals including humans, which in natural course stops with menstruation or defilement. They also acknowledged the influence of the moon as evil and the source of menstrual cycles, which with the data already given tends to show their elders understood the basic tenet of our Vitalogical Sciences.

They had a secret language, esoteric knowledge and a history dating back 8,000 years at Blavatsky's time speaking of events 187 generations ago, when they arrived from the Land of the Sunrise bespeaking of Pre-Adamite conditions in Paradise. H.P.B. did penetrate deeper in their mysteries conversing with their elders. As to the after-life of their people, they said, "Their bodies become forage on the mountains which the buffalo eat. But the love of our children and our kinfolk becomes transformed in fire that ascends to the sun, and there it blazes eternally with a flame that gives warmth to our buffalo and other Toddes." The Solar Fire is composed of the Fire of Love, expressing warmth of the heart well. Not only the Toddes' love, but the love in every one who is good, living as they do, becomes the Light and Warmth giving Life to all in the Sun, they added. These people with a pre-history dating back to when the buffalo were considered sacred companions of a frugivorous race, thus must antedate the Aryan migrations from the north accompanied with more domesticated cows, horses, etc. and their amalgamation with the black racial tribes of Southern India, as represented in the Krishna and Gopi traditions. The small black Kurumbu tribe of black magicians were sickly and cadaveric and smelled evil, making tangible their use of animal and prey they lured hypnotically to capture. The most numerous were the Baddagues, who were muscular, medium stature, ate fruit, roots and grains, dealt with the outside world and maintained a status as Brahmins among other tribes. H.P.B. quoted various writers before her, altho these tribes are fairly unknown outside of India, and her work was published in Russian, thus delaying this disclosure.

Studying with Swami Sivananda's Reshikesh Yoga Vedanta Forest University, and others, milk and fruits are taught as the ideal Sattwic Diet for the practice of Yoga. However, we do not recommend the use of fresh milk, impregnated still with animal nature, but rather the bacterial culture of plant growth after it has been transformed in a ripening process, free from pasteurization, antibiotics, pesticides and other modern forage toxins, and of sacred surroundings in animal kindness in milk storage.

Like Elaine Pagels says in "The Gnostic Gospels", "some Gnostic Extremists agreed with certain radical feminists who today insist that only those who renounce sexual activity can achieve human equality and spiritual greatness.", meaning that giving birth, sex losses, are sins the same as killing.

Of the children born to the Toddes, only one out of four were females or "mothers" as they called them. This is an idealistic proportion even for Vitarians,- avoiding motherhood. This compares with the teaching in the "Gnostic Gospel of Thomas" saying a woman must become a man, or not bear children in continence, for Spirituality. We have thus even considered the idea that the homage that the Toddes did to their buffalo was somehow an esoteric veneration to an early Buddha: Turning the two "ff"s in buffalo inverted, we have "Budda-Lo" or shall we say the "Loka" or Plane of Buddhahood!

Why did the Toddes only allow those living without defilement or menstrual and seminal losses, to milk their buffalo and watch over the storage vats in a Spiritual Devotion that absolutely no one else was allowed to witness? We know that milk can be contaminated with the wrong type of aerial bacteria, just as it can be turned into wholesome food by friendly bacteria (by enzymatic action). If stored with onions, or other vegetables, milk will take on their flavor, altho most disagreeable to us would be milk stored near slaughtered flesh, or in toxic aluminum containers. Leviticus chapt. 15 of the O.T. Bible treats seminal and menstrual losses, and objects in contamination with the same, as well as such persons coming in contact, under specific rules about defilement, which speaks for some Esoteric Essene Teachings being retained therein even now. It shows lusty lives were contagious like milk bacteria. Vitarians have also found this contagious influence among people who have sex losses: Unless one lives among those who have no losses, the holy, it becomes hard to maintain purity (in body, mind and soul). The relationship of milk and sexual contamination among us, the Toddes and mention in religious scriptures indicates the existence of a Sacred Science of Sealing the Sex. Continent saintly people are known to give off a heavenly fragrance, fruitarians (of long standing practice) smell like the fragrant fruits or their blossoms, healthy people radiate health, and spirituality radiates in luminous auras." (unquote M.M.M. 1981)

Human milk at the time of an infant's greatest increase in growth, doubling its weight in 6 weeks, contains only 1.6% protein, very similar to juicy fruits, altho of the highest class of proteins. Vegetable proteins are also high class proteins, altho more abundant than in fruits, while milk curds are much like vegetables since they are derived from grass or green vegetation. All of these have enzymes that make their assimilation into the blood without further digestion necessary after they have been masticated and mixed with the saliva and swallowed into the stomach.

However, the curds must be used only in small proportion of about one tenth of a large mixing bowl of salad, giving the correct balance in a low protein proportion to a high living water percentage. That mixed omnivorous people thirst while eating, liking to wash down their food with milk or other beverage, shows they naturally feel a lack of living water and nutritional enzymes such as found in fruits, vegetables besides concentrations in milk curds which balance with living water. Thus large bowls of salad made of choice greens mixed with one-tenth portion of curds, cottage cheese, etc. will supply the minimum protein requirements of a much higher quality, but with the necessary enzymatic action, and without enzyme inhibitors disturbing their metabolism.

A calf builds more bone in a year than a human in a lifetime. In turn, an infant builds more brain in a year than a cow does in a lifetime. Yet cows, goats, sheep, deer, mares, buffalo, reindeer, camels and other green vegetation eating animals have been used for human food since time immemorial. Human milk contains about half the calcium of cow's milk. Then again we note that collards and kale have twice the calcium of cow's milk. Limes, lemons, oranges and berries have equal the amount of calcium that human milk contains, which is true of carrots, celery, head cabbage, leaf lettuce and a great portion of salad vegetables. Our use of curds and cheese is only justified if one's intestinal digestive enzymes are lacking, and provided that only a small one tenth proportion to a large mixing bowl of salad is used, altho elderly persons may have a greater proportional need than one-tenth part. As to the symbiotic relationship of man and his cows, goats, etc. in our chemically disturbed world, there are many objectors called "Vegans" who use absolutely no animal products, yet they liberally use avocados that are specifically fertilized with dried slaughterhouse blood, but may be labelled "organic" as a fertilizer, which in principle supports the meat packing industry. As early Hygienists pointed out, animals are unable to produce any kind of food, the food substance in dairy products thus being valued as green leaf protein, collected for human use by symbiotic partnership with milk giving animals in exchange for their own sustenance with pastures. As soon as cows and milk animals are fed grains and dozens of modern substitutes, our green herb principle for food along with fruits is violated, and can be justly criticized. Graham and his followers used milk for numerous years and found it unnecessary, as such, not realizing that milk like fruits must be matured for mature adults to provide a natural plant source of food supplementary to salad vegetables made necessary by modern conditions in life on earth. Yet, unlike other Hygienists, we usually reject the use of seeds which lack nutritional enzymes, being replaced by reproductive enzymes, which overload the human economy with reproductive substances causing sex abuses, or is a basic source of crime, population excesses, war, and the world problem syndrome. However, since Dr. Shelton and his Hygienic predecessors recommend the use of cottage cheese, along with the use of nuts which we avoid generally, we find it convenient to base our teachings on their pioneering work on Hygiene. See Dr. Herbert M. Shelton's "HYGIENIC SYSTEM, VOL. II ORTHOTROPHY" as a basic text.

Before going on further with our own Vitalogical Hygiene, let us include Shelton's 9 Rules for:

CORRECT FOOD COMBINING:

(1.) Never eat carbohydrate foods and acid foods at the same meal. (Fruit acids prevent carbohydrate digestion and favor their fermentation.)

(2.) Never eat a concentrated protein and a concentrated carbohydrate at the same meal. (Dr. Richard Cabot of Harvard said: "When we eat carbohydrates the stomach secretes an appropriate juice, a gastric juice of different composition from which it secretes if it finds proteins coming down.) (3.) Never consume two concentrated proteins at the same meal.

(4.) Do not consume fats with proteins. (Fat inhibits the proper flow of gastric juices to digest proteins, but the fat-starch combination is good for the stomach and the intestines.)

(5.) Do not eat acid fruits with proteins. (Nuts and fresh cheese are about the only protein foods that do not quickly decompose under such conditions and these have their digestion delayed. Lemon, lime juice and vinegar check hydrochloric secretion)

(6.) Do not consume starches and sugars together. (Sugar and starch cause fermentation when taken together..)

(7.) Eat but one concentrated starch food at a meal. (It causes over-eating.)

(8.) Do not consume melons with any other foods.

(9.) Milk is best taken alone or let alone. (We use no fresh milk,-curds or cottage cheese are just as essential in needing ripening as are fruits.)

If you find yourself choking or with nausea wanting to vomit, while eating a salad with organic green vegetables, and these were washed with chlorinated city water, this is due to an over-dosing of chlorine, an "inorganic" acid-forming mineral, which is poisonous. Steam escaping from radiators using chlorinated water is known to cause death, just as soldiers were killed in World War I with the same gas. Your editor never drinks water, only using fruits and vegetables containing Living Water and their juices so as to never thirst. At least one should have a charcoal water filter to avoid poisoning organic carrots, etc. for juice and salad vegetables washed in such poisonous water that destroy the body's enzyme secreting faculty.

When we insist on the correct enzymes in food, this applies emphatically to certain soy-meat loaf, soy-burgers, nut-roast or cutlets, and other flesh imitations or substitutes concentrated in proteins, which are really another junk food foisted on the unwary public. First soy oil is chemically extracted from soybeans, so that such oil has no enzymes for its metabolism. Then the by-product known as soy flour or meal is likewise with harmful residues of the chemical used, beside being an anti-enzyme reproductive substance denatured in the process. That a cup of soy flour contains 42 grams of protein mean little if the body is unable to assimilate it. Snake venom is pure protein, but in that very fact it is poisonous to the human bloodstream. One of the good points Dr. Shelton brought out about the mind, was that "One of the most indigestible things in the world is the human mind. Once a man lets his mind in his stomach he is sure to have indigestion of a chronic character". Many of us have developed prejudices against certain foods later to discover that such foods may have been just what we needed.

Our first publisher, Dr. J. D. NARULA of Delhi, India lived to be 115 years old in 1978, when the newspapers celebrated the event with front page headlines. With the help of our teachings in his latter years he was able to prolong his life on to the super-centenarian level when your writer was making the centenarians of Vilcabamba famous. When we had another subscriber to our teaching, Dr. Zinn of the Canary Islands, visit him in 1974 he confirmed the following facts at the age of 111 years: Dr. Narula's diet consisted mainly of fruits and clabbered milk, fresh green peas and papayas. He drinks carrot juice and rarely eats cooked vegetables or chapatis. He considers bananas too starchy, preferring apples, and hardly ever eats almonds, which he believes is the only alkaline nut. He avoids all acid formers in bulk. We quote Dr. Gerhard Zinn Ps.D. or to use his Eastern name, Hatha Yogi Sri Brahachari Vishnu Premi, as we describe in Transcendent Truth Teachings: "His son of 75 years looks much older than he with 111 years of age. Dr. Narula still has grey hair mixed with black ones at the side of head whereas his grandson of 40 is all white. None follow the old man! He received his Doctor of Naturopathy in U.S.A. 50 years ago... In Yoga philosophy he showed only full ignorance disclaiming well known masters in India and so on. (Having understood our teaching, many now ignore Yoga which is a cover-up for wrong diet, which makes problems of over-propagation, hunger, disease, while government researches in nuclear weapons, pesticides, etc.) (Unquote) Dr. Zinn had several interviews with Dr. Narula. Dr. J.D. Narula published our books on "Spiritualizing Dietetics, Vitarianism" and "Modern Live Juice Therapy" under the trade name of C. T. Hospital as the publisher. This was followed by "Omangod Press" of Dr. Viktoras Kulvinskas who published the same in the United States.

Dr. Zinn also visited Swami Sivananda's Ashram at Reshikesh, and to explain his corpulence, said: "Of course Sivananda gave up Sadhana, and eating more food, got that fat as you know it, living only on cooked food, but he will not have had any sex losses consciously or unconsciously," going on to defend 8 or 10 hours of Sadhana (rigorous Yoga exercise just to avoid fat, and avoid eating right! Yet the mainstay of Indian Ashrams is pulses, chapatis, rice, etc. Our recommendation that Dr. Zinn visit Mt. Abu Jains who William Goodell reported about as living on a handful of figs each day and living to be 1,200 or 1,400 years old, with hair trailing behind them on the ground, of which Goodell showed us a documentary report with a picture of one who was 750 years old, was replied with: "I had to cancel my visit to Mt. Abu since conditions in India nowadays are that people have to eat what they can get," and told of the lack of toilets, filth and poverty preventing further travel. Vitalogical Hygiene prevents what takes 8 to 10 hours of Sadhana to undo.

VITALOGICAL HYGIENIST
AGAINST BIOLOGICAL SCIENCE CATEGORY

We cannot call our Science Biological Healing or Hygiene because Biology teaches that Life is a biochemical or a biophysical attribute, or both, and Life evolves from a chance spontaneous generation from nothing. Moreover, the ignorance of the Living God, or the meaning of "Jesus" (Yeshue) as we translate the Scriptures, that is the God of Life, threatens the very Life of our planet. The Theory of Darwin's Evolution that texts on biology are based upon, was schemed to oppose the tyranny of the Church authority, but however righteous this was, it obliterates the Omniscient Creator, Designer and Order that regulates Life at all times without the chaos of chance happenings. This was brought out by H.G. Wells, who wrote in his famous "Outline of History" as to the teaching of Darwin's theory of Evolution: "A real demoralization ensued. There was a great loss in faith after 1859. Man they decided is merely a social animal like an Indian hunting dog... Two World Wars followed. Every year manifests greater beastliness of man as an animal, subjection and limitation is daily imposed on our young at school, with mass realizations of crime and war, as well as human life destruction with man's inventions in medicine, agriculture and industry. Only when man manifests his higher Intelligence by working with lower forms, have animals improved in species. Otherwise their Force, Direction or Intelligence is limited to Form." (unquote, H.G. Well's attack was formidable)

When we quote or refer so often to Dr. Herbert M. Shelton's Orthobionomics or Natural Hygiene, which he defines as a biological science, it is because of this category it is unanimously accepted as the science of the evolution of life in these limitations set by Darwin and his successors, and not as simply as the Science of Life. Shelton was a difficult "on-the-fence" fencer, who fended, or offended both sides of the opposite lots. In his Hygienic Review, Oct. 1970 he deplores, "If only we could open the eyes of biologists so that they may recognize pathology, they would soon discover that nature is full of pathological developments that they have mistaken for evolution. The greater part of the scientific world today centers its concept of evolution around mutations, of what used to be called sports or freaks of nature." Again on March 1971 he wrote, "Applying recapitulation theory to the baboon and taking the skull and face as our measuring rod, the baboon is descended from man. This is plainly evident from the fact that a young baboon closely resembles man in skull shape and facial formation, while the adult baboon more closely resembles the dog in these same particulars. It may be that we have been reading the process of evolution backwards. Instead of having man evolve from some ape-like ancestor, man would appear to be the progenitor of apes as was suggested by Mivart." To the other side of the fence we see Dr. Shelton's constant classification of man among the primates, the anthropoids; especially the gorilla as well as the chimpanzee, meaning man's diet should be like theirs, frugivorous, consisting of fruits, succulent herbs, to which he adds nuts. Yet, the facts are that nuts are not found in the environment of these higher anthropoids, the only exception being coconuts, the most ideal among nuts for its low protein content, which is believed to be the food of the small monkey, while the squirrel and other rodents like rats show how nut eating pathologically devolved anthropoids into stunted creatures. Likewise, the grain-eating Indians of the Andes are a 4 foot statured race. The use of curdled milk products, sourkraut and other vegetables besides rye bread among the tall Scandinavians, Russians, Finns, etc. like our description of the Toddes who lived on curds and fruits, shows how diet greatly affects human stature and health. The 3 foot Kurumbu tribe of flesh eaters showed the contrasting features that devolved humans into beastly creatures from a race like the Toddes, none of which were less than six and a quarter feet tall, who in turn had descended from even more godly ancestors.

Dr. Shelton said he was often asked, "Who made you God?", when he insists his instructions must be strictly followed. We have seen how certain people adhere to Yoga with beliefs that 8 or 10 hours of Sadhana remedies all man's troubles, or spontaneous generation of life by evolution and a chance "big bang" did away with a need for God, and similar errors, yet if they followed the early Hygienists, it would be found that Creator was the Source and the Science of Life. "The Spirit is Life-Giving, the body is of no profit." (Jn.6:64)

"BERAESHITH" is the first Word in the beginning of the Bible, the translation of which is "At-first-in-Principle" or the "Archetypal" of the Creation made by the Elohim. The Elohim made man in their own image and likeness, that is, an archetypal prototype, or the Heavenly Man. Thus the Son of Man spoken of in our Gospel who comes in the clouds of heaven is the Son of the Heavenly Man, Anthropos of the Bible's mystical anthropology. This Creative Word is the Fountainhead of John's Gospel, Epistle and Apocalypse, each of which begin with a tribute to the Word of God as the Word of Life, or the Son of Man, Anthropos or the Image and Likeness of God, the Father or Godhead. "But there had stood in the midst of you one whom you do not know... A Man who came before me, is in my Presence and shall remain after me." (Jn. 1:26,30) This Man, Anthropos or Adam Kadmon, is the Prototype of the Spiritual Man that was made by the Elohim, in the Image and Likeness of God, or Androgynous.

Androgynous means both male and female in one, hermaphroditic. He was the Life that was the Light of men, and thus the Light of the World, for all things were made by Him.

From this it can be seen that evolution came into theoretical scientific speculation because men had become blind (Jn.1:5) as to seeing the Light in the Book of Life depicted in Johannine Scriptures. So John's "Jesus" is the ideal Spiritual Man, Omnipresent and Eternal, that is only known by spiritual experience, coming in the clouds of heaven as he describes in his Revelation, altho present among his true Apostles in this life midst those who experience Him who was the Word in Prototype. The use of the Word to describe the Scriptures, in the Wisdom teachings, as well as the Logos of Philo of Alexandria, and the other early Greek writers as to fulfilling the Essene ideal. The Aramaic root is in "Meloca" refers to angel, messenger in being, and not just a mortal human person. Fullness or the Plenitude is the Pleroma of Gnostic speculations.

For those preferring a scientific perspective, physics holds that the atom is the small dense nucleus having a positive electric charge of 1 to 92 or more (depending on the kind of atom), and 1 to 92 or more electrons surrounding in concentric shells. From this it is obvious that what has been taught in the East for millenniums, or that all matter is a sensual illusion, or Maya, reflections of light, sound, touch, smell and not the real thing itself. The universe is an illusion created by two small lens in the eye. Matter is ultimately etheric, consisting of theories about electrons and positive charges, or fictitious invisible reflections. Things do not materialize, because everything is spiritual, altho the mind gives us the illusion of materialization, limitations, impenetrable matter and other fixed attributes.

Unfortunately the nineteenth twentieth century materialism searched for exact sciences and values, and thus became established on all kinds of false theories as we have shown about spontaneous evolution, pharmaceutical medicine, chemical stability and such fallacies. When Dr. Shelton taught Natural Hygiene as a biological science of Orthobionomics, we do not infer that he was deluded in terms of the science of his early twentieth century knowledge, but when he tried to penetrate into the realms beyond the Maya of modern physics, he made statements that were really negative and ignorant in fields beyond his materialistic mind.

There were other Hygienists and Orthopaths who disputed his claims. Dr. Gerald Benish of Escondido, California promoted iridiagnosis as a hygienic practitioner who contributed articles regularly to Dr. Shelton's Hygienic Review, many others unlike Shelton believed in the use of enemas, colonics and other methods, while Art Andrews, a Hygienist of San Jose, California founded a Religion of Natural Hygiene, in spite of Dr. Shelton's view that religion was evil. Likewise Dr. Shelton inferred that not only were my teachings the polar opposite of Natural Hygiene, but that Natural Hygiene was neither spiritual, metaphysical or mystical. In other words, he opposed Jennings, Graham and Trall, the chief founders of Hygiene who based their teaching on Vitalism and the Bible.

Now, it is evident that Graham, and especially Shelton, depend on their intellect which is based in false assumptions, and not in the Divine Wisdom of the Elohim. Man was not created in the image and the likeness of beasts (Apoc.20:4), or the primates: He was made in the Image and Likeness of God. Worldly Science, according to the prophecy of the Evangelist John, would lead man into the worship of the likeness and image of the beast, as has happened with the theory of evolution, which fathered man on an ancestry of beasts. The fact is that during the glacial ages when men took to living like the beasts, eating their flesh and dressing in their skins, he took on beastly characteristics of the carnivore, or granivore he paid homage to. That is why the devil is pictured with horns, hooves, the tail and other features of beasts aggregated to the gross human attributes. The grosser that human food becomes, the grosser his body becomes: The more ethereal or invisible substance of elements he takes on, such as hydrogen, oxygen, nitrogen and carbon dioxide gases in likeness he transforms himself, escaping into the ascension of being thru superconsciousness, free of the animal corpse he took on in his Karmic wanderings. Foremost, we must forget the worship, or intimate knowledge of the Science of Good and Evil taught from the devil's Tree, which is deviltry, in the image and likeness of the beast, and become fashioned in the likeness and image of the Elohim, the Creative Gods. "The souls of them that were beheaded for the testimony of Jesus and for the Word of God, and who had not adored the beast nor his image nor received his character in their forehead (intellect) or on their hands, who shall live and reign with Christ a thousand years."

Neither Graham nor the other early Hygienists, as well as Shelton had any idea of the real source of Hygiene as given in the original Bible Scriptures, since only in the most recent research of translation are the names of the authors among various Gods revealed. The first chapter of Genesis claims to be the Word of God, the Elohim, who existed before "Yahweh", the name of the tribal God of the Hebrews or Israelites. Such people claim to be the followers of the God of the Covenant, or Old Testament, which is an alliance Yahweh made with them at Sianai, allowing vicarious atonement, or substitute animal sacrifice for the sins of these Hebrew-speaking people. Obviously, from the first chapter, Genesis deals with man,

Anthropos, as an androgynous being, or both male and female, without the animal method of reproduction. Because the American Hygienists never discovered what the Tree of Life and the Tree of the Science of Good and Evil consisted of, they ate both of the juicy fruits and their dry seeds or nuts, saying they were both fruits. However, the first chapter distinguishes clearly that the juicy fruits and the succulent vegetables were the food of man, and the seed they yield for the reproducing of their own kind was for their respective purposes, and thus not for nourishing man. When man consumes juicy fruits it gives him life, because it contains living water with food enzymes that cleanse and regenerate man's vitality. When he eats dry seeds or the reproductive material of plants, therein he only obtains reproductive enzymes for growing new plants, and not for human cellular replenishment enzymes needed for health, and like slaughtered flesh of animals, only have the degeneration and death programming traits of their substances to provide in attributes. Had the translators of the Bible been real Hygienists, they would have perceived the meaning of the first chapter of our Scriptures as the handbook for the layman in understanding human health. Dry nuts made man dry up with age.

Elohim, who in the second chapter guides man is supplanted with "Yahweh-Elohim", whom the Yahwist Hebrews have vested interests in. In the third chapter, sin is introduced by the serpent, and woman becomes pregnant, and man has to toil with sweat on his brow to grow more reproductive substance, grain for bread in a vicious cycle, because they sinned eating seminal substance of plants rather than from the tree of life or living eternally. We must remember, Like begets like, not unlike.

The fourth chapter story of Cain and Abel, is wholly "Yahwistic", since Elohim is not mentioned, and both the grain grower Cain and the shepherd Abel, make sacrifices of their produce to Yahweh, announcing the birth of the Yahwistic cult of the Israelite Hebrews in vicarious atonement. The Essenes did no homage to Yahweh, showing why it is so important we know which God is being worshipped, since when John refers to "In the Beginning" or in the Prototype of the first chapter as the archetypal model, later he will refer to the Serpent as a liar form the beginning, leading man astray into delusion and sin in life. The Essenes and the Gnostic Christians or Nazarenes refused to do homage to the tribal God, Yahweh, who demanded animal sacrifices, showing why they rejected many or the majority of the books of the Old Testament for their Scriptures. The Latin and Greek Church translations completely cover up such differentiations, altho the word God is used usually to mean Elohim, and Lord is used to refer to Yahweh, yet the Bible-reader is ever under the impression that the two Gods are the same. This is like calling Satan and the Son of God

Spiritual Beings, which is true but for opposite reasons. In John 8:42 he says: "You are of your father, the devil, and the desires of your father you will do. He was a murderer from the beginning and he stood not in the truth, because truth is not in him. When he speaks a lie, he speaks of his own; for he is a liar and the father thereof." Thus, John clearly classifies these Jewish Yahwistic followers of Abraham. In Matthew 21:43 states plainly to the Jewish Elders and priests: "The Kingdom of God shall be taken away from you, and shall be given to the people yielding the fruits thereof." Yet, the obscene and unholy teachings of many of the books of the Old Testament were foisted upon Christians as the very inspired Word of God altho the primitive Essene Nazarenes, or Gnostic Christians rejected them.

To the materialist, the Ascension into Spirit is an absurdity. Yet, when a man is tired at night or is sick, he must lay down on a bed to recharge himself, just like the hour-glass must be shifted to reverse the flow of sand gravitating to earth. To rise against gravity, after sleeping at night, or after an illness man must abstain from heavy, earthy food, such as grains, legumes, nuts, seeds and flesh, that is, everything that depends on earthy gravity like death. Fasting on organic H_2O or water, the living water of fruit or vegetable juices, or even eating juicy fruits, will bring back health quicker than taking any earthy food or water that the beasts struggle to survive upon, altho they fast when sick by instinct. Eating of the mistaken, forbidden fruit that the devil prescribed, man became like the fallen angel, Satan, or "gods" in the knowledge, desire or science of the intellect. The intellect is based on grasping and craving of the senses, which altho it may acquire the whole world, it only brings gravity to the dust, the earthy matter from which it was derived. Not only the Bible, but the Buddha, the source of the Essenes, taught the same truth.

While the Essene Gnostic interpretation of the Serpent is to "learn by Divine Experience" (as Browne-Landon also interprets it), the Yahwistic Jewish interpretation would remain to be to "learn by worldly experience". Thus, today the translation read, "The woman said, The serpent beguiled me". But who has ever seen a talking serpent? Thus, what is meant, is that the teacher from whom Eve learned to eat of the forbidden fruit was the worldly mind within her, or the intellect that reasons by sensual experience or desire. The Tree of the knowledge of good and evil, is also translatable as the Tree of the Desire to know Good and Evil, and since "Eden" means Desire which is in the midst of the garden, it locates the garden within one as the garden of pleasures or desires of the senses. Now the Intellect, built on worldly experience of the senses, is what leads to evil, but the Divine experience of Spirit is Good, Beneficent or Spiritual Joy in Consciousness.

There are various ways to reflect on these mysteries. One may see the brain reflected by peering into the obscure black darkness at night, and placing a candle below one's line of vision about one or two feet from the face, while slowly moving the flame back and forth to the sides a foot, and the form of the brain will be seen even in a person with no spiritual training. In turn the forbidden fruit of the Tree of the Desire to know Good and Evil is obviously found in nut trees especially, since when cracking pecans, walnuts, etc. the united kernels resemble the male and female or androgynous human brain by listening to the deviltry of intellect, desire to experience good and evil.

The worldy intellect, based on sensual desire has analyzed millions of bits of knowledge as to the minerals, vitamins, amino acids and other food factors, only to betray one to the sensual desires. After abandoning the medical drug physicians, many health enthusiasts become walking encyclopedias on nutritional necessities, that is, profound intellects centered on self-medications, obtained now from Health Food Stores, or Natural Pharmacies. In their homes, in their pockets, in their automobiles, etc. they have collected a miniature replica of their Health food Store. Since their intellect is established on the health virtues of all kinds of substances, a whole array of vitamins, desiccated liver, bone meal, amino acids, seaweeds, dolomite, dried fruits and vegetables, etc. So they never stop craving and eating one thing or another to establish a balance, since such things with additions of each new concentration give a new unbalance that has to be remedied. Thus, it was no wonder that numerous writers about the supplementarily health foods necessary for perfect health died before the average life span of 70 years, such as the case with J. I. Rodale, while persons living simply of fresh fruits and vegetables and their juices, such as Dr. Norman Walker live as he did 127 years, (publisher's note: his actual age is unclear, some saying 109 years, others 113, others 127) or double the life-span of the heavy concentrated supplement takers. Each food satisfaction makes for another corresponding deficiency in elements to balance it, indefinitely. The easiest way to end all this hankering is to finish one's meal with some food most abundant in living water, yet having the least in calories or other concentrated food factors, such as carrots, zucchini, cucumber, chayote, kohlrabi, etc. or slice of a papaya or an apple.

This Garden of Eden down in the depths of the belly nourishes the Serpent of Desire of the sensual intellect, and likewise has lead many dietary neophytes little by little to nut or seed eating, cooked foods, etc. until they are back on their former flesh eating and narcotics consuming habits. After Noah and his family survived the Flood, like Abel made an altar to sacrifice their first-born clean animals, which records the first surgical intervention prescribing certain rules on incision and bleeding in the name of Yahweh, the God of Vicarious Atonement. The Yahwistic Religion and Medicine identify, not only in the surgery of animals and bloodshed in destroying the enemies of these tribal conquerors, but likewise the use of narcotics, especially alcohol, along with similar pain-relieving drugs. Thus, Medicine is born along with surgery as an aftermath of eating forbidden food in Eden.

The Serpent was more subtle than all the beasts of the field that Yahweh-Elohim created. Subtle means mentally acute, given to or characterized refinements of thought, insight perception and analysis. Subtle, crafty, artful and keen is the associated definition of Webster's, and thus the caduceus or Mercury's staff with serpents entwined became the symbol of the medical profession, remedying the Serpent of Edenic Desire in the depths of the belly, assisted by the crafty intellect. In turn, the Vitalogical Hygienic System is based on the first chapter of the Bible's Genesis, and ends with John's esoteric writings interpreting the same in the final New Testament Scriptures. Thus, it should be mystically, metaphysically and spiritually based on Divine Experience only perceived by spiritual meditation, rather than matching wits in crafty and clever arguments and reasoning in the talking serpent of sensual desires, the pleasures born in the Garden of Eden. The more we dwell on and analyze foods, the more attached and illusively held by the fascination of the beast and its image we become by this crafty devilty of Eden's Serpent. By placing the thought in the Realm of Heaven, the Presence of God, the Spiritual and Vital Powers in man transmute the grosser elements into ethereal being, the Elohim, Sons of the Living God, Jesus and the Buddha.

Many who fasted at Dr. Shelton's Health School, he admitted, spent their days talking only about food, so one sees how attached to their source of evil pleasures in foods they remained. The next step would be an intellectual fast, living on fruits and vegetables, but abstaining from mental nutritional feasts, by dwelling on the Almighty Presence of Divinity within which is the Source of Living Joy. "Whosoever is born of God, committeth not sin, for his seed abideth within him, and he cannot sin because he is born of God. In this the sons of God are manifest and the sons of the devil". (I-Jn.3:9) This refers directly to God's Plan in Genesis, in that eating only juicy fruit and succulent vegetables, with the "living water that springs up into Life Everlasting", we live in perfect continence, not desiring nor knowing sexual indulgence, giving birth to children not born of God, and the degeneration of the race beyond our means of restraint. But eating seeds one has seminal losses, menstruation, brain and nerve depletion giving attachment to food and sexual gratification, the sons of the devil of beastly reproduction just as did the primates that in time devolved from Eve, the mother of all the living.

Thus the first chapter of the Holy Bible is the Divine Design for the way of life and what should be food of the holy person, the Son of God, showing that only those food, fruits and vegetables are omnisciently prepared by the God of Creation, to contain the highest living water proportions coupled with the exact enzymes for direct instant assimilation, the right proportion of protein, to the calcium and the phosphorus content, and all the necessary dietetic factors. No human, no matter how learned about nutrition can keep in health as well as the all knowing Creator who designed human beings and the correct foods for him. As we have shown, those considered authorities on nutrition do not live as long and as well as ordinary people ignorant about nutrition and only the raw food eating vegetarians are enabled to live super-centenarian lives, while the Paradisian diet without seeds taking only the fruits and succulent herbs enables lives nearest to a millennium in years. However, without engendering children even this might be extended indefinitely.

Yet, your writer did not discover the principle of seeds being the forbidden food, or degenerative factor along with flesh eating, by reading the Bible. Actually, it was due to his conscience, the intuitive Word of God speaking within the human heart and genes, that he decided not to eat other sentient beings like himself, becoming a vegetarian before he was able to intellectually defend his actions. Then due to failing eyesight, partially due to his search into the lives of others who chose to live as he did, he consulted a Naturopath in Seattle since he had been advised to stop studying so much, skipping a year in high school.

The Naturopath treated him with infra-red and ultra-violet ray lamps, electro-magnetic massage, and gave him some wheat and rice germ to take as a prescription. However, the wheat and rice germ immediately gave him copious seminal losses, very obviously proving to him that it was the reproductive principle that is found in all seeds that is contrary to the consumer, and it can seriously deplete his organism of nerve and brain building substances. Altho, your writer was never accredited with these findings in the mid nineteen thirties, he later learned that Dr. Edward Howell had made the same discoveries on his own, and is now accredited as America's pioneering biochemist and nutritional research-er into Enzyme Nutrition and contrary effects of enzyme inhibitors, or anti-enzymes. Continuing his research after graduating from Kirkland High School in 1938 when he had adopted an exclusively fresh fruit diet, in a couple of occasions that he was forced to eat walnuts, or almonds, the same thing happened as with the wheat and rice germ use back in 1936, so he began teaching that in fact any nut and seed eating in general was contrary to the health and integrity of humans, similar to eating animal flesh.

Thus it was 1944, or 8 years later, that reading the Holy Bible, I discovered that the God of my conscience and intuition, had also been teaching this same principle, since the Elohim had proclaimed this very principle as the First Precept taught to man. Vitalogical Sciences were thus gloriously founded by the Elohim whom made man in their likeness an image in the beginning of time in the beginningless past!

However, altho the Holy Bible may contain the essence of the God in-spired teachings of the Essenes, Nazarite-Nazarenes and John the Baptist, Evangelist and Apostle taught, yet like many other works of men the same collection of books, also contains an assortment of pornography, obscene and decidedly devilish precepts which John and his Spiritual Guide, Jesus, condemned. Like the early teacher, Marcion and his fol-lowers proclaimed, the Hebrew portion of the Bible contained both the teachings of the Good God, the creator of the Prototype spiritual man, as we have illustrated as Elohim, and the mischievous Evil War God Yah-weh, who was the God of the Old Testament believers in cruel sacrificial rites of Vicarious Atonement who taught rape, homicide, slavery, looting, deception, and similar immorality simultaneously with pretexts of foster-ing the commandments of God. Both the Old and the New Testament, tell of the followers of the true God Elohim, and the supplanters, who come in the guise of Yahweh-Elohim in the second chapter of Genesis, but by the fourth chapter have led men into immorality.

Now, Dr. G.R. Clements, Dr. Walter Siegmeister and other writers on Virgin Birth claim that man was bisexual, or a hermaphrodite with a normal physical body of flesh just like everyone today, which representation may be understood erroneously. However, they say the female is superior, and will become the bisexual super race of the future, seeks to remedy the perverted erroneous interpretation. In Genesis 6:4 it states: "When the Sons of God came unto the daughters of men, and they bore children with them, the same became the mighty men of renown, and Yahweh saw the wickedness of man was great on earth, and that every imagination of the thoughts of his heart was only evil continually." Thus, we see that the Sons of Elohim of the first chapter of Genesis, "were made in his own image, in the likeness of the image of the Elohim he created them". (1:27) But in it we see the nature of Adam, and Seth who were given sons in the spiritual image and likeness of the Elohim. The race in the likeness of Elohim were androgynous, but when the woman Eve and the serpent led man into sin, Yahweh-Elohim said: "In the sweat of they face shall thou eat bread till thou return to earth, for out of it wast thou taken, for dust thou art and into dust shall you return" Likewise, Yahweh makes a covenant with the Yahwists that he "shall not destroy man because the inclination of his heart is evil from his youth (8:21) Yahweh, after receiving animal flesh offerings promises not to cut off all flesh by the Flood (9:11) showing the evils that the flesh of man is heir to.

The Sons of God, the Elohim, are those who live in absolute continence conserving their seed, and are born again of the Spirit of the Divinity and living water, according to John's teaching. Thus the Sons of God live on fruits and vegetables, but the sinners in an aftermath to eating the forbidden food, were given the herbs of the field and bread eaten in the sweat of the face, (3:18), which gave them male and female flesh in the nature of earth, being clothed with human skin (3:24) As we have sought to illustrate, the Sons of the Elohim were a Spiritual Race, living in the Presence of God, while the earthy man with their hearts inclining to evil, live centered in a flesh-born body clothed in sentient skin, the medium of sensual pleasure. As Clements illustrates, rabbits and other animals are known to give birth by Parthenogenesis, so Virgin Birth of human flesh is like that of such devolved animals, and not the true Androgynous Sons of God like the Elohim

The God Presence in Many like the Elohim, is still One in Spirit, so the plural is thus singular, and vice versa, so John says, "Ye are Gods, and still speaks of giving us "the power to be made Sons of God to those who believe in his Name". (Jn.1:12) Consequently, as a corollary to the last paragraph, God is male, the Father, Son and Holy Spirit, in primitive

Christianity, Father, Son and Mother were considered the Trinity, just as the earliest versions of New Testament acknowledge. Only a life dwelling perpetually in the Presence of God will enable one to live on juicy fruits especially, and even perhaps including vegetables in most cases. But if seeds, nuts and especially cooked grains or bread are included, the life span is reduced to 120 years. (Gen. 6:3)

This explains why the Bible's patriarchs before the Flood lived 900 years, more or less, but the earlier they began to eat bread and beget children, the shorter was their life span.

However, when Noah worshipped Yahweh, sacrificing and eating animal flesh, and planting vines he drank wine to quiet his conscience from his guilt for committing sin in killing, this led to the rapid degeneration of the race. It is noteworthy that the age of Cain and his Yahwist grain-growing and eating descendants are not recorded, so as to show their insignificance, while the followers of the Elohim, like Seth lived nearest to a millennium. "And Yahweh said, My Spirit shall not strive forever in man, for that he also is flesh, yet his days shall be a hundred and 20 years." (Gen.6:3) The Bible's story so well known to people educated in the religious tradition thereof, depicts the virtues of Spiritual Hygiene in the image and likeness of the Elohim, and the Sons of God are an excellent exemplar for our Vitalogical Sciences.

SCIENTIFIC PRINCIPLES OF
VITALOGICAL HYGIENE AND RELATED SCIENCES

The Vitalogical Sciences have found it most instructive to flesh born humans to compare human food with naturally basic human nutritive attributes of mother's or human milk. The high levels of minerals to protein, with 75 to 95 percentage of living water, considers more or less about 2% protein as ideal, altho some greens and olives we accept as excellent in over 4%. Kefranyr of Max Planck Institute found a complete balance of nitrogen and performance ability can be maintained on 25 grams of protein, and Oonian and Hipsley studied people in full health, magnificent muscular structure and physical performance on only 15 to 20 grams protein daily. Sherman criticized the 70 grams protein specification of early 20th century as an erroneous high protein mentality. Vitarians have proven it successfully and raw foods greatly reduce the amino acids one needs for health giving portions.

In basic principles, as to the self-healing power of the body, per se this is a myth, because this would mean dead corpses could heal themselves since they too are bodies. Rather one should say Life is self healing, since all healing is achieved by Life, an attribute of the Living God. We have already explained the Vitalistic principles. This is why Vitalogy teaches all healing is with Life, and the greatest "Health Food" which the Living God, Jesus, taught, (speaking thru John) was living water, which "springs up into Life Everlasting". This is why we need 80 to 90% or more living water in whatever is food as found in what the Living God, among the Elohim taught as God-Given Food in Genesis 1:29: "And the Elohim said: Behold I have given you every herb bearing seed upon the earth, and all trees that have in themselves fruits that yield seeds of their own kind, to be your food", just as in 1:11 states: "And the Elohim said, Let the earth bring forth vegetation, the herb yielding seed after its kind, and the fruit tree yielding fruit after its kind, where is their seed, upon the earth; and it was so. This illustrates that: if the herbs and fruits, that are our God-Given food, yield their seed after their species for their propagation, then using seed as a source of our food is forbidden by their inherent true purpose.

The late Dr. Bernard Lytton Bernard, in a report in "Let's Live" magazine, shows that ordinary well, spring or earth water is inert, stagnant or dead water, requiring 13 or more days for he body to expel it, unlike living water with enzymes, vitamins and minerals that insure hygiene in the cells of the whole human body. This 13 day dead water stagnation was proven by electronically tagged water molecules. The burden is complicated by the presence of limestone, iron oxide, salt and other dead inorganic minerals in earth water making such water pathologically adverse to the kidneys and liver functions. Dead earth water is to the body, like what atheism of modern science is to the Spirit of man. From the first the Hygienists, as well as Dr. Shelton in recent times, insist that inorganic water is the only liquid that should be drunk for thirst, being against the taking of fruit juices.

As we brought out in "Modern Live Juice Therapy" in 1962, living water from fruit and vegetable juices both nourish and satisfy thirst and hunger being essentially one and the same need for man's true food, thus being a feeling of a need for juicy fruits and later succulent vegetables, or their juices felt in the flow of saliva and dryness of the throat. This is because living water contains enzymes that enable its immediate assimilation by the blood, beside enzymes enabling the removal of waste from the cells in every part of that body beside enzymes for the mineral, amino acid, carbohydrate and fat assimilation into a recuperative effort of the renewal of life. No wonder that John in his Gospel speaks the Word of the Living God, Jesus, to the woman at the well in Samaria, saying he would instead offer her living water springing up into Life Everlasting.

At the so-called Wedding of Cana he served the guests grape juice just pressed from fresh grapes, who said he had reserved the best new wine to the last, since this is the total cellular replenishment felt thru-out the human constitution partaking of living water, a daily internal baptism of living water and Holy Spirit. In turn, drinking inert dead water, without enzymes that give Life and being to living things, one takes on an unwanted burden to the system, that instead of being a daily cleansing, makes the body balk in having to accept, unable to remove for two or three weeks, hampered by watery deposits of inorganic liquid. Moreover, the 1% mineral matter of earth water contains corrosive or caustic iron rust, limestone, salt and other inorganic minerals that fill the body with deposits that harden the arteries, and the body tissues in general, beside making the bones brittle with osteoporosis, and makes every movement of the body painful with the oncoming of old age and invalidism. As in the eating of bread and grains man returns to the dust of the earth, so also drinking water in 40 years man takes within himself enough limestone to form a full sized marble statue of his body. Dr. Shelton's ignorance as to living water and its functions, claiming there is no such thing, like his advocacy of nuts and seeds really lacks the comprehension of our Buddhist Essene Gospel of Jesus, beside the most modern science of enzymatic living water nutrition we promote in Vitalogical Hygiene for complete vibrant human vitality, beside burdening themselves with anti-enzymes that inhibit the realization of an everyday baptism with living water that springs up into Life Everlasting in the Holy Spirit.

One of the more progressive theories of science admits advisedly that everything in nature is intelligently designed for its purpose, sometimes called biological purposefulness. Herein we have an easy accommodation in that each enzyme has its special purpose, and thus the nature of its purposefulness must be respected for true Vitalogical Hygiene and Health. Fruits and succulent herbs had their purposefulness as food for man, and their respective seeds had purposefulness in the propagation of their own kind, so consequently when reproductive enzymes are used for food they are inhibited in action, or anti-enzymes contrary to their purpose. Jesus is the Life-Giving Spirit, meaning the Living God, just like the Creative God(s), the Universal Life of all, which spoke thru the Evangelist, John. Let Jesus live, move and have His Being in you. In Him is Life and the Resurrection into Life Everlasting.

Dr. Bernard Lytton Bernard also brought out another factor in the atrophy of the function of the liver, in a report from J. J. Parker and Jan Siemenson of the University of Southern California, which held that if the liver had been removed or severely injured by an accident, it still may be regrown. It shows that a Vitalogical dietetic regimen on organic foods can be used to flush out and restore a newly regrown organ. The reason why old age and disease can come about is because the liver cells are clogged or destroyed with wastes which atrophy their function. Lack of hygiene, high acidity, cholesterol, calcareous and uric acid deposits fill the body with the ailments of old age. Chemical fertilizers especially attack the liver function, destroy cellular respiration and the Vitamin A supply.

Fruits and vegetables are man's natural diet, and thus are a highly alkaline source of Vitamin A. In turn, cod liver oil and other fish liver oils are highly acid forming sources of Vitamin A, which nullify their benefits. The golden or orange colored fruits and the green chlorophyll containing herbs are the richest sources of Vitamin A of the most alkaline types of foods, enabling the regrowing of the liver cells and body regeneration.

The myth of complete proteins being found in animal proteins is basically due to herbivorous animals living on grass. Thus, dairy products are elaborated from green grass, and animals are completely incapacitated in synthesizing proteins which is exclusively the function of plants. In England where grain eating has been abused, vegetarian scientific research came to the rescue. Since grasses supplied the food elements needed by the body, they went to the source of superior proteins in plants. And that is what they found, even greater quality in grass and green leaves in general. Leaf proteins are superior and have more amino acids than grains and other seeds. What makes leaf proteins superior to seeds and animal products is the highly alkaline attributes, and the enzymes required for their digestion are present. The British made "Plant Milk" from vegetation. Now they get their food elements direct without 90% waste of food values lost in maintaining animals in life and health. We hope this research will continue elsewhere, altho in the meantime our symbiosis with cows still ensues.

A number of eminent writers have held that cancerous growth is accelerated by the acidity of the blood due to the diet, and alkalinity of the blood prevents the formation of cancer, as was supported by Dr. Alexis Carrel. In turn Vitamin A maintains the health of the mucous membranes or epithelial cells, as the anti-infection vitamin, this being where cancer usually forms.

As to infection, the electron microscope, according to "The New Microscope" by Dr. R. E. Seidel and M.E. Winter, tell us that ten different classes of germs exist only, but within each class, taking on new forms by altering the environment and food supply... harmless benefactors such as colon bacillus can be turned into deadly typhoid germs. Dr. Royal

Raymond observed that, "If the metabolism of the human body is perfectly balanced or poised, it is susceptible to no disease", and it is only the chemical constituents of these microorganisms acting upon the unbalanced cell metabolism that actually produces the disease. R.M. Newcomb in 1951 reported that with the 17 varying bases of media, from lemon juice to putrid liver, 17 varieties of germ life were brought about. Dead matter like body waste, and toxic chemicals are the only food that germs can thrive upon. This proves the teaching of the Vitalogical Sciences which declare, man produces his own disease organisms from friendly human benefactors, by feeding on toxic substances. By observing correct cellular hygiene eating the Vitarian diet, we do not feed disease. Excess or unbalance in good food can also become toxic.

Since it is proven thru radioactive tracers that 400 grams of protein is daily synthesized by the body, just as it is autolyzed in a fast, only a small percentage is needed to replenish the supply. We actually destroy our protein supply by eating in excess of the minimum requirement of fruits and vegetables, coming from the toxic destruction of cells. Human milk has only 1.2 grams of the 400 grams that are synthesized by the body. All the amino acids are formed in the body's 400 gram reserve, so how can anyone lack any except in long term imbalances of inferior proteins. Fingernails grow while one fasts, without needing protein from food. This is why wounds of the body heal faster when one fasts.

We have spoken of Living Water content as a basic factor in identifying the Natural Vitalogical Diet. By this we rule out all unnatural combinations which are not living foods. Food preserved in glass jars or cans often imitate our low protein, high water content, but chicken, beef, noodle, tomato and vegetable soups are very far form being Vitalogical foods, even if they mimic their portions of water, protein, minerals, etc. in cases. Likewise, Dr. Shelton's Hygienic menus using nuts are not correctly balanced. He has said there is no food factor in vegetables and animal products that is not also available in fruits, but in this he includes the forbidden fruit, which is actually the seed or nuts of trees to supplement fruits or as a single food in the diet. At the end of this topic, we shall give you a DIET CHART for our DIETETIC SCIENCE OF CHASTITY out of which we select Vitarian foods that contain about TWO PERCENT PROTEIN in the natural uncooked state when picked. Our diet is not a man-made kitchen concoction, or even a food chemists nutritional combination, but rather how nature, or our Creator, compounded its only intended food for man, without additions, adulterations or other alterations. After such alterations, chicken soup has 1.4% protein, cooked farina has 1.3% protein, corn grits 1.2% protein, and altho these are ideal protein percentages, yet none of these are Vitarian foods. We also recommend some foods above the 2% protein level such as calcium-rich greens, leafy vegetables, herbs and dried fruits so there are more factors to consider rather than just low protein percentages. It is easy enough to reduce the protein percentage of any food with a pitcher of water, or by cooking in water, but we refer to the LIVING WATER CONTENT of cellular composition in contrast to Low Living Cell Protein Content. A baby grows to double its weight in six weeks on less than 2% protein, so the key to health among humans rests in such low protein percentages. The other factor that controls the desirability of some Vitarian foods over others, is the CALCIUM CONTENT IN PROPORTION TO THEIR PROTEIN CONTENT. Altho fruits average as rich in calcium as mother's milk, some people think of them as poor bone-building foods, when really they are the nearest semblance to what makes babies bones and teeth grow healthily so fast. Another vegetarian, a former chemist, writes: "Seeds and nuts are necessary to the vegetarian diet. Few vegetables and fruits contain enough calcium. I got a set of chemicals for urinalysis and to my great surprise I lacked calcium myself and I eat seeds." Now, this man unwittingly agrees with us. He eats seeds and does not have enough calcium in him. Before going further, how can one determine calcium deficiency by the urine, when normal findings are on a very perverted diet. People are getting enough earthy inorganic mineral calcium, but are unable to benefit their health from it since it is hardening the body tissues rapidly, and yet they are starving for living calcium that can make the tissues elastic and youthfully durable.

The purest quality of food would build cells lasting the longest, since toxic foods and the resulting cells wear and tear the body down fast, which accounts for the cleanliness and lack of sediments in the urine on the fruit diet.

Now, those who think seeds have a lot of calcium, should notice that corn flour has only 6 milligrams (mg.) per 100 grams or about one fourth pound of flour. But corn has 8 mg. or 8 times the needed protein to balance the calcium. So naturally there is only less than one milligram of calcium to each gram of protein, and needs 50 times over the amount of calcium it has! Raw wheat has the 40 mg. of calcium like mother's milk, but has 12 times the needed protein, so it needs 400 mg. of calcium, or 10 times more for the same calcium-protein proportion as human milk.

Seeds, or reproductive matter, augment the reproductive fluids of the body pathologically cast off by the body, dividing what minerals we have, for the "sexually adequate" feeling mistaken for strength. Eventually in old age the reproductive function gives out, so the lime and other alkaline substances are needed to neutralize the excess acidity of the protein intake. Man becomes saturated with calcareous lime and earthy deposits, while the flesh acidity burns with irritation and pain, - actually a potent chemical factory but biologically lacking life to move it.

Two of the tallest boys I knew who grew up as life vegetarians on grains, nuts, legumes and other seeds beside cow's milk, as well as the fruit and vegetables Americans enjoy, yet despite their long bone structure, they had bad teeth. They wondered about their neighbor's boy who grew up eating mainly on candy and sweets on a very bad diet, and yet had perfect teeth. Some of us see this occur here and there, but there are many other factors to be considered. At least their long bone structure could be accounted for by the excess calcium in milk, since here in the high Andes originally the Indians lived on barley and corn without milk and vegetables practically, and they were a race only of about 4 feet in stature. Even if the calcium content of some foods is high, if the protein is proportionately 10 times too much as we illustrated above, the excesses of protein consume the usable calcium present to fight off the destructive blood acidity coming form excess protein decomposition, and moreover, mines the calcium out of the bones and teeth to produce healthy reproductive fluids. This makes for an excess of homosexuals, crime motivated rape, beside the unbalances in health in bones, teeth, nerves, brain, organs, etc. that seem hard to explain by limited dietetic factors. Actually the 40 mg., or .04% calcium of human milk is beyond our needs as adults theoretically: an infant's body and bones increase very rapidly and thus need, but with less needs in adults, we could do with half as much, just as there is only half the need of protein found in human milk. The great stumbling block is the consuming of excesses in protein in flesh and seed foods in most civilized countries which destroy the calcium reserves of the body. Some claim citrus fruits destroy the teeth because they lack calcium. This is untrue. Oranges for instance have exactly as much calcium as human milk, 41 mg. to a 100 gram portion. Ripe oranges with most of their peel have 70 mg. calcium to 100 gram portion. Limes and lemons have 33 and 26 mg. calcium respectively, while tangerines have 40 mg. calcium for 100 gram portion like mother's milk.

The best sources of calcium are to be found in garden greens, or green leafy vegetables. Collard leave have 250 mg. per 100 gram portion, Kale 249 mg., turnip greens, 246 mg., parsley 203 mg., dandelion greens 187 mg., broccoli 103 mg. Thus greens are our most concentrated food proportionally in calcium, while the fruits and other vegetables contain more or less the amount of calcium in proportion to their protein in closeness to human milk. Now, altho we do not wish to confuse our students, there is one exception to our seeds lacking in calcium category: Sesame seeds, whole, contain 1160 mg. calcium to 100 gram portion but then they have 18..6 grams of protein in a 100 gram portion, 966 times as much as human milk. Other seeds also have high calcium portions such as almonds with 234 mg., soybeans 226 mg. filbert 209 mg., Brazil nut 186 mg. and chickpeas (garbanzos) 150 mg., all of which have excess protein to calcium proportions. Another source of high calcium proportions are seaweeds,- Kelp with 1093 mg. calcium to 7.5 grams protein, dulse with 296 mg. calcium to 25.3 grams protein, which are near the garden greens protein-calcium proportions, altho not having ideal living water content, and should be de-salted (soaked in pure water) to avoid sea salt excesses.

The calcium in fruits and vegetables is not a second-hand food, already used for body cells as is the case with animal flesh; needless to say fruits and vegetables have the correct portions of protein, minerals, vitamins, and enzymes for their assimilation and molding human cells. To give the bloodstream a used carcass to build new cells from is like giving a mason used mortar or concrete, containing the minerals necessary for a construction, but not in usable form. It is as useless as old used cement. Farm animals fed on grains age and die more rapidly due to calcification of their tissues. One of the richest foods in calcium (altho not proportioned to its protein) is Swiss Cheese which contains 27.5 grams of protein with 925 mg. calcium in 100 gram portions: it lacks little only to the calcium-protein proportion of human milk. Here again as with dried seaweed, dehydrated green vegetables and fruits, etc. there is a need to compensate for the lack of living water with fruits or vegetables low in calories but with high living water content.

Another factor to be aware of is that the inner bleached leaves of such vegetables as lettuce and cabbage contain much less calcium than the outer green leaves, which in the case of lettuce may have only 20 mg. of calcium for Iceberg lettuce, while in the case of Cos Looseleaf lettuce that does not head up and bleach the calcium content is 68 mg., over triple, whereas the protein content per 100 grams is the same. But it may be objected by some that mustard, turnip and other such greens which are doubly rich in calcium, are too hot or not appetizing in the raw natural uncooked state, except in minute quantities. The least damage to the enzymes and vitamins, and the most natural preparation of food is by drying or dehydration which can happen in an open field to both fruit and vegetables. Vegetarians use a great amount of dried fruits, organically grown in the U.S.A. Our first clue as to the higher calcium proportion offsetting a little more protein we mentioned in "Spiritualizing Dietetics,-Vitarianism" diet chart, noting that the higher alkalinity of dried olives, even with 4% protein gives a Vitarian (sexual fluid conservation) reaction. Olives are doubly richer than human milk in calcium, so dried they are over half a dozen times richer in calcium than mother's milk. We have stressed the living water content of the diet as a positive aspect of Vitarianism, and restricted 2% protein generally (other than greens), but if we take in large proportions of living water with extremely low protein portions such as in apples, watermelon, chayote, cucumber, lettuce, etc. the calcium to plant protein proportion is a better guide.

People coming on to our Vitarian diet have often been tempted away even after healing of menstruation or seminal losses, by health food propaganda that proclaims they are not getting enough calcium, etc. Yet these are the very calcium depleters of the human body that they should be avoiding, since they are building up excesses of seminal substance from foods which give sexual losses and lay the ground for all ailments that prosper from overfeeding.

The hot California sunshine in a couple of days will leave freshly picked greens so dry and crisp that they can be powdered between the fingers, altho elsewhere it may take a couple of weeks. Anyone, anywhere can avoid the intense heat of cooking by simply oven drying (with the oven door open, comfortable to the hand) of greens and fruits, and this is one of the many things a sauna may be adapted to do, unless one has a special electrical food dryer. Leaving a little circulation with the low heat tolerable to cellular life like one does in sunbathing, much of the excess perishable fresh fruit, garden greens and wild herbs can be preserved for times of the year they are not available. After dehydration pass the leaves thru a screen or sieve and the powder or flakes can be stored in jars in the case of greens or herbs, or whole in case of dried fruit. The mentioned mustard and other piquant greens take on a salty cheesy flavor delightful for salads, dried basil, dill, etc. being specially nice, avoiding the use of salt-laden seaweed, or even worse salt that harms kidneys, eyesight and gives adipose flesh.

However, the greatest precaution must be observed in the case of green leafy vegetables and herbs in that they should be dried in the shade, avoiding the direct sunshine, since that bleaches and destroys the green chlorophyll, beside injures the flavor and food properties. However, in removing the living water by low heat dehydration, we must be conscience clear of returning the living water balance with high living water content foods, or fruit and vegetable juices consumed slowly well insalivated as a living food or a food for Life.

Perhaps, it is vain to hope that others avoid our pitfalls using a transition diet, since many never get out of such a rut, or even fall back worse. The next best treatment for food increasing the flavor, altho it crosses over to killing heat temperatures which destroy the enzymes beside some of the vitamins, if not the usability of some minerals, is to be found in baking or steaming vegetables in their own juices in a waterless cooker. Altho an iron pot may be used, stainless steel is better, with an inner dish that is slightly (1/2 inch) above the bottom, which can be filled with artichoke, endive, kale, cabbage, squash, etc. which will give the foods a natural salty flavor, often provoking the desire to drink vegetable or fruit juices later in the day. However, remember you cannot coerce the Creator by adding water or fire to food to make it right as a substance for building healthy human cells. He originally ripened fruit for man's perfect food, and whenever we need minerals, enzymes and other factors we have green vegetables. If you must use water, the earthy minerals should be filtered out using pine resin crystals, or distilled water is best. We would prefer our students avoid such compromises, because living water rich raw living food contains enzymes and life energy that empower the brain and nervous system to make one's own will coincide with the Will of God, who is Almighty, the molder of Gods among men.

Finally, the high calcium proportion to the protein guide in the Vitarian reaction of foods explains why greens are best with double the protein of the 2% borderline foods such as potatoes, avocados, etc. Potatoes and avocados contain one-fourth the calcium content of mother's milk to the same protein proportion, and yet they have 4 to 5 times the phosphorus proportion to their calcium, which we shall see is also calcium consuming.

Phosphorus releases food energy, or assists in the metabolism of carbohydrates. Here it is not how much again, but what proportion. The phosphorus content of our choice are neither high nor low, altho they seem to account for a need to supply man's superior brain and nerve development. The juicy fruit diet usually supplies half again as much phosphorus as they have calcium, these superior brain foods including apples, apricots, grapes, mangos, peaches, tomatoes, watermelons, etc. Berries, celery and carrots have an equal balance, while cabbage, greens, figs, olives, all citrus fruits, etc. have more calcium than phosphorus, so as to be more body or bone builders.

As such, phosphorus by itself is not a brain food, since the most degenerate brain, chickens fed on grains, are the most stupid and neurotic, to which many grain fed persons resemble, and are constantly being deprived of their egg or seed substance faster also. Yet in wheat there is 35 times the phosphorus to its calcium content, in corn there is 29 times as much, while fish and meat have 17% times more phosphorous than calcium. All seed and animal flesh being over 10, 20, or 30 times too rich in proteins likewise for human consumption.

BESIDE EXCESS PROTEINS, ANOTHER CLUE TO EXCESSIVE REPRODUCTIVE FLUID FORMING SUBSTANCE IN HUMANS IS THE EXCESS PHOSPHORUS CONTENT. Wheat germ with 1118 mg. pumpkin and squash seeds with 1144 mg., sesame seed with 616 mg. soybeans with 554 mg., Brazil nut with 603 mg., black walnut with 570 mg. and almond with 504 mg. in their phosphorus contents are far beyond comparison to mother's milk with only 10 mg. of phosphorus content, only one one-hundredth part or one fifth part in the case of almonds. Apples have 10 mg. phosphorus, nor do you find cauliflower with 72 mg. too high in relation to the calcium and protein proportions. According to Victor Lindlahr, EXCESS PHOSPHOROUS DESTROYS THE CALCIUM UTILIZATION, which may also account for the small frame or stature of seed grain eating people like the Andes Indians who live on corn mainly with 178 mg. to 6 mg. phosphorus to calcium ratio. Other grains, legumes, nuts and seeds with hundreds of milligrams of phosphorus give excesses which along with the acidity of their excessive protein destroy or consume the calcium, giving seed eaters bad teeth and bone deficiencies.

Now, we have mentioned sour milk products, curds and cheese as being similar to fruit in needing to be ripened, milk animals really living on the greenest of greens having abundant chlorophyll, so that in the symbiotic relationship to man, they provide the essence of plant enzymes and green leaves in their milk. Unlike, grains, seeds and the flesh of animals, the calcium to phosphorus, protein to calcium ratio resemble the ratio of green vegetables. Cow's milk has 3.5 grams of protein, 118 mg. calcium to 93 mg. phosphorus. Goats in same ratio have 3.3 grams protein, 129 mg. calcium and 106 mg. phosphorous. So taking broccoli we have 3.3 grams protein, 130 mg. calcium and 76 mg. phosphorus, and in collards we have 3.9 gram protein, 249 mg. calcium and 58 mg. phosphorus. Dandelion greens are eaten by man and cows, which also have 2.7 grams protein, 187 mg. calcium to 70 mg. phosphorus ratio, while cabbage has 1.4 grams protein to 46 mg. calcium to 31 mg. phosphorus ratio. But when cabbage is dehydrated it has 14 grams protein, 394 mg. calcium to 288 mg. phosphorus ratio. Thus, comparing dehydrated greens with higher protein grams, and calcium to phosphorus milligrams ratio in Swiss cheese produced from milk curds resembles the dehydration of greens in these ratios, Swiss cheese having 27.5 grams protein, 925 mg. calcium to 563 mg. phosphorus.

Yet, unlike the case of dehydrated greens in which a great deal of the enzyme potential is destroyed by drying, in turn according to Howell and enzyme researchers, Swiss cheese and other forms of cheese are of the highest enzyme digestive power. As long as the calcium ratio to phosphorus is higher the catalytic power in foods seems to be benefited if the source is of man's natural food in herbs and fruits beside the symbiotic dairy products derived from herbs.

Continuing the study of other minerals, we always come back to CALCIUM, THE KING-PIN, or the hub of the wheel of life to which all other elements must conform in right relationship. The nitrogen or protein must be in right proportion to the calcium as in human milk, the phosphorus next, followed by iron, and then the magnesium, beside some other minerals, are known to destroy calcium utilization in their excesses, and vitamin D and others for their lack. Cooking alone also destroys up to 72% of the calcium in cabbage, and 32% of the calcium in other vegetables on the average. Dr. Sherman has said that abundant calcium would add more years of life, and other nutritionists have made a cult of calcium by attributing to it a remedy for all ills nearly universally. This is quite all right, if they are not getting excesses or have no lack in other minerals, vitamins, enzymes, amino acids, or other factors that do not cancel their utilization. The right proportion to a relatively low proportion of protein is likewise necessary, altho such foods like Swiss cheese, dried alfalfa powder, etc., are of exception since the original food they were derived from was relatively low in amino acids.

An illustration worthy to note is that beet greens are a very rich source of calcium (119 mg. per 100 grams) but used cooked, the excessive 3.3 mg. of iron has been shown to actually de-calcify the body. Your editor was tempted into using oxalic acid vegetables rich in calcium and iron, cooked without water because of their salty flavor to dress his raw salads about 1960 in Otavalo, and a severe oxaluria. The calcium in his body was being lost as calcium oxalate, becoming rickety, anemic and dia- rrheal. It was stopped by cutting out beet greens, Swiss chard, spinach, etc. and using more alkaline vegetable salads raw such as lettuce, cabbage, carrot, cauliflower, etc. Similar difficulties come with other calcium-deprivers. Finally, let us observe that fruit is the only food our Creator made pleasant to behold and delicious to eat thereof as given in first precept to man in the Bible. A child instinctively, naturally and surely intuitionally craves sweet fruits, altho the parents mistakenly try to feed the acid-forming pap made of cooked grain and animal flesh in their false prejudices. Heavy protein foods like animal flesh, legumes and grains are acid forming requiring salt, chocolate, coffee, tobacco, and other alkaloids to balance them in cravings, and thus a vicious cycle starts without end trying to balance one craving with its opposite. A wiser course would be to live as our Designer made us as to diet.

==

NATURAL VITALOGICAL DIETETIC CHART
GIVING BASIC RATIOS IN FOOD ELEMENTS

==

PER 100 GRAMS: Compared with "Composition of Foods" by U.S. Dept. of Agriculture Handbook, "Composition and facts about Foods" by Ford Heritage Researcher, etc.

EACH FOOD IS LISTED IN THE FOLLOWING ORDER FOR EACH NUTRIENT OR CLASSIFICATION CATEGORY:

FOOD WATER PROTEIN CALCIUM (P)PHOS. IRON CLASSIFICATION (RAW)
HUMAN 87 gm 1.2 g.   40
mg.   10 mg. .2 mg. Enough calcium &   MILK   or %   or%
                                  protein to double in   1 or 2 months
after birth   weight   in 2 mo.
                                                                JUICY
FRUITS

Food	Water	Protein	Calcium	(P)Phos.	Iron	Classification (Raw)
Apples		84.8 g.	.2 g.	7 mg.	10 mg.	.3 mg. King of fruits
Apricot fresh	85.3	1.0	17	23	.5	Vit. A, Copper
Apricot dried	2.0	5.0	67	108	5.5	Brain food (Phos)
Avocado	78.0	1.3	10	42	.6	Ideal Salad dressing

111

FOOD (RAW)	WATER	PROTEIN	CALCIUM	PHOS.	IRON	CLASSIFICATION
Banana com.	75.7	1.1	8	26	.7	Energy food
Banana red	74.4	1.2	10	18	.8	Eat alone
Banana dryed	3.0	4.4	32	104	2.8	Tropical treat
Blackberry	84.5	1.2	32	19	.9	Eat w/ banana creme
Blueberry	83.2	.7	15	13	1.1	Cal.-Phos. ratio good
Cherry sweet	80.4	1.3	22	19	.4	Iron sugar rich fruit
Cherimoya	73.3	1.3	23	40	.5	Rich energy fruit
Date	22.5	2.2	59	63	3.0	Extra rich sweetness
Fig fresh	77.5	1.2	35	22	.6	Ideal to live on
Fig dried	23.0	4.3	126	77	3.0	Use soaked
Granadilla	75.1	2.2	13	64	1.6	Gives variety
Grapefruit	84.4	.5	16	16	.4	Excels tree ripe
Grape Con.	81.6	1.3	16	12	.4	Grape diets are
Grape Euro	81.4	.6	12	20	.4	Cleansing, energizing
Husk-Tomato	85.4	1.9	9	40	1.0	Quick growing fruit
Guava com.	83.0	.8	23	42	.9	Rich in minerals
Lemon peeled	90.1	1.1	26	16	.6	Living water rich
Lemon peel	87.4	1.2	61	15	.7	combine with other
Lemon juice	91.0	.5	7	10	.2	citrus juices
Lime	89.3	.7	33	18	.6	Limes are more alka-
Lime juice	90.3	.3	9	11	.2	line than lemons
Loquat	86.5	.4	20	36	.4	Tropical apple juice
Mango	81.7	.7	10	13	.4	A tropical favorite
Olive Mission	73.0	1.2	106	17	1.7	Calcium rich

FOOD (RAW)	WATER	PROTEIN	CALCIUM	PHOS.	IRON	CLASSIFICATION
Orange peeld.	86.0	1.0	41	20	.4	Calcium rich
Orange juice	88.3	.7	11	17	.2	Short juice fasts
Papaya	88.7	.6	20	16	.3	Tropical enzymes
Peach fresh	89.1	.6	9	19	.5	Brain, nerve building
Peach dried	25.0	3.1	48	117	6.0	energy fruit
Pear	83.2	.7	8	11	.3	Rich in fruit sugar
Persmon. kaki	78.6	.7	6	26	.3	Alkaline sweet fruit
Pineapple	85.3	.4	17	8	.5	Tropical fruit king
Plum	81.1	.5	18	17	.5	Best fresh
Pomegranate	82.3	.3	3	8	.3	Wonderful juice
Pricklypear	88.0	.5	20	28	.3	Use darker kind
Raisins	18.0	2.5	62	101	3.5	Great energizer
Raspberry blk. rich	80.8	1.5	30	22	.9	Mineral
Raspberry red	84.2	1.2	22	22	.9	Excellent
Strawberry berry food	89.9	.7	21	21	1.0	Quick
Tangerine favorite	87.0	.8	40	18	.4	Citrus
Tomato ripe	93.5	1.1	13	27	.5	Fruitarian choice
Tomato juice	94.0	1.1	7	15	.4	Rich food & drink
Watermelon	92.6	.5	7	10	.5	Wonderful diet

SUCCULENT VEGETABLES

FOOD (RAW)	WATER	PROTEIN	CALCIUM	PHOS.	IRON	CLASSIFICATION
Artich. Jerus.	79.8	2.3	14	78	3.6	Use grated in salads

FOOD (RAW)	WATER	PROTEIN	CALCIUM	PHOS.	IRON	CLASSIFICATION
Artich. Globe	85.5	2.9	51	88	1.3	Favorite vegetable
Asparagus	91.7	2.9	22	62	1.0	Wild in old gardens
Beet red	87	.3	1.6	16	.7	Used for tumors
Beet greens	90.9	2.2	119	40	3.3	Calc. rich raw
Broccoli ite	89.1	3.6	103	78	1.1	Another favor (contains starch)
Brussel Sprt.	85.2	4.9	36	80	1.5	Grate fine in salad
Cabbage Chin	95.0	1.2	43	40	.6	All cabbages are great
Cabbage Crn.	92.4	1.3	49	29	.4	salad base, even make
Cabbage Red	90.2	2.0	42	35	.8	sourkraut without salt
Cabbage Sav.	92.0	2.4	67	54	.9	are economical organic
Carrot	88.2	1.1	37	36	.7	Tender whole or grated
Cauliflower	91.0	2.7	25	56	1.1	Author's favorite (starch)
Celeriac	88.4	1.8	43	115	.6	Rich in calcium, phos.
Celery	94.1	.9	39	28	.3	Mineral rich
Chard Swiss	91.1	2.4	88	39	3.2	Cooked gives oxalur.
Chayote	91.8	.6	13	26	.5	Great juice extender
Collard leaf	85.3	4.8	250	82	1.5	Richest calcium greens
Collard lf/ste	86.9	3.6	203	63	1.0	Excellent in salad
Corn sweet	72.7	3.5	3	111	.7	Eat fresh on the cob
Cucumber	95.1	.9	25	27	1.1	Excellent in salad

FOOD (RAW)	WATER	PROTEIN	CALCIUM	PHOS	IRON	CLASSIFICATION
Dandelion	85.6	2.7	187	66	3.1	Rich in minerals, alka.
Escarole	93.1	1.7	81	54	1.7	Blood alkalizer greens
Fennel	90.0	2.8	100	51	2.7	Rich juice, easy growth
Garlic	61.3	6.2	29	202	1.5	Leaves best, dressing
Kale leaf	82.7	6.0	249	93	2.7	Very rich in calcium
Kale lf./stem	87.5	4.2	179	73	2.2	Use for salad minerals
Kohlrabi	90.3	2.0	41	52	.5	Eat like apple or salad
Lettuce Bibb	95.1	1.2	35	26	2.0	Favorite salad base
Lettuce Cos	94.0	1.3	68	25	1.4	note loose leaf have
Lettuce Icbrg.	95.5	.9	20	22	.5	> minerals than head
Turnip greens	90.3	3.0	246	58	1.8	Rich in calcium

VITARIAN SUPPLIMENTS

FOOD (RAW)	WATER	PROTEIN	CALCIUM	PHOS	IRON	CLASSIFICATION
Milk cow's cultured	89.0	3.5	118	93	.1	Clabber salad dressing
Milk goat's	87.4	3.3	129	106	.1	Clabber dressing
Cheese cottage	76.5	19.5	96	189	.9	Fresh Curds
Cheese Swiss	39	27.5	926	563	.9	Rich Enzyme food
Cheese Ched.	37	25.0	725	495	1.0	Enzyme rich food
Whey	93.2	.9	51	53	.1	Excess Lactic Acid
Mung sprouts	88.8	3.8	118	340	7.7	Enzyme for starch
Soy sprouts	86.3	6.2	48	67	1.0	Enzymes, low calc.
Wheat grass						Enzymes, for juice
Alfalfa meal	7.4	22.7	349	73.5	13.0	Mineral concentrate

FOOD (RAW)	WATER	PROTEIN	CALCIUM	PHOS.	IRON	CLASSIFICATION
Cabbage Dry.	4.0	14.4	394	288	4.9	Calcium rich

SEEDS, NUTS, LEGUMES, GRAINS NON-VITARIAN FOODS

FOOD (RAW)	WATER	PROTEIN	CALCIUM	PHOS.	IRON	CLASSIFICATION
Almond	4.7	18.6	234	504	4.7	Enzyme inhibitor
Barley	11.1	8.2	16	189	2.0	Calcium poor
Bean Lima	10.3	20.4	52	142	2.3	Alkaline bean
Bean Mung	10.7	24.2	118	340	7.7	Use sprouts only
Bean Pinto	8.3	22.9	135	457	6.4	Use sprouts only
Bean Fava	11.9	25.1	102	391	7.1	Anti-enzymes
Bean fresh	72.3	8.4	27	157	2.2	Avoid use
Brazil nut	5.6	14.3	186	693	3.3	Protein Anti-Ezymes.
Cashew	5.2	17.2	38	373	3.8	Toxic anti-enzymes
Coconut meat	50.9	3.5	13	95	1.7	A nut
Corn flour	12.0	7.8	.6	178	1.8	Calc. poor, indigest.
Garbanzo	10.7	20.5	150	331	6.9	Use green or avoid
Lentil	11.1	24.7	79	377	6.8	Enzyme inhibitor
Millet	11.8	9.9	20	311	6.8	Anti-Enzyme cooked
Pea green	78.0	6.3	26	116	1.9	Eat like green corn.
" dry	11.7	24.1	64	340	1.6	Anti-enzyme cooked food
Peanut w/sk.	5.6	26.0	69	401	2.1	Acid-forming anti-enzyme
Pecan	3.1	9.2	73	289	2.4	Anti-enzyme tempter
Rice brown	12.0	7.5	32	221	1.6	Anti-enzyme, cooked food
" white	12.0	6.7	24	94	.8	Starchy cooked food

FOOD (RAW)	WATER	PROTEIN	CALCIUM	PHOS.	IRON	CLASSIFICATION
Oatmeal	8.3	14.4	53	405	4.5	Anti-enzyme raw or cooked
Rye	11.0	12.1	38	376	3.7	" " " "
Sesame whole	5.4	18.6	1160	616	10.5	Anti-enzyme raw food
Squash seed	4.4	29.0	51	1144	11.2	" " " "
Sunflower	4.8	24.0	120	837	7.1	" " " "
Soybean	10.0	34.1	226	554	8.4	Excess protein, phos.
" fresh	69.2	10.9	67	225	2.8	Sprouts best, emergency
Walnut Black	3.1	20.5	trace	570	6.0	Acid-forming anti-enzyme.
Walnut Eng.	3.5	14.8	99	380	3.1	" " " "
Wheat	12.5	12.3	46	354	3.4	Acid forming, cooked food
Wheat germ	11.5	25.6	72	1118	9.4	Strong aphrodisiac.
Chicken growth	71.2	20.1	14	200	1.5	Artificial hormone
Eggs	74	12.8	54	201	2.7	Unborn chicken, low calcium
Beef	47	22	9	158	2.8	Unnatural grain fed
Cod	82.6	16.5	10	194	.4	Jesus's disciples are the Gospel's fish, he eschews fish, fowl and flesh foods.
Halibut	75.4	18.6	13	211	.7	
Lamb	66.3	17.1	10	191	2.6	Jesus condemns eating lambs.

FOOD (RAW)	WATER	PROTEIN	CALCIUM	PHOS.	IRON	CLASSIFICATION

SLAUGHTERED FLESH, FISH AND FOWL

FOOD (RAW)	WATER	PROTEIN	CALCIUM	PHOS.	IRON	CLASSIFICATION
Liver Pork	72.3	19.7	10	362		
Pork	50	14.1	8	151	2.1	Both Jews and Moslems never eat unclean pork
Salmon	63.4	17.4	--	289	.9	

NON-VITARIAN PSEUDO-RATIOS IN SOUPS:

FOOD (RAW)	WATER	PROTEIN	CALCIUM	PHOS.	IRON	CLASSIFICATION
Beef soup	91.6	2.4	6	25	.2	Soups imitate water and protein ratio of fruits, and even calcium to phosphorous ratios.
Chicken soup	93.1	1.4	8	8	.2	
Noodle "	90.4	2.4	33	34	.1	
Pea soup	86.2	2.6	13	40	.6	Man can never create the life-giving en zymes of true "living water" in real "living food".
Tomato "	90.7	.9	10	16	.4	
Vegetable	91.6	1.7	13	20	.3	

BREAD, DRIED AGAINST OVEN BAKED

FOOD (RAW)	WATER	PROTEIN	CALCIUM	PHOS.	IRON	CLASSIFICATION
Carob meal	6.3	7.7	22	1	.5	High calcium to phos. ratio, St. John's Bread; Mashed banana/carob flour.
Graham Crkrs	5.5	8.0	20	203	1.9 bread	Graham's hygienic
Swedish Crsp	6.5	12.4	50	400	4.4	Swedish "health" bread.
Szekeley	13.4	13.6				germinated wheat wafer what Szekeley called his "Essene Bread' made by soaking wheat, grinding and sundrying.

| W. wheat brd. | 36.6 | 9.3 | 96 | 263 | 2.2 |
| White bread | 34.5 | 8.2 | 65 | 81 | .6 |

Some hygienists eat a little whole wheat bread Vitarians eschew it, and white bread is chaotic.

COMMENTARY ON ABOVE DIET CHART

==

We tried to give an unbiased listing of foods eaten in the world today, starting with our recommended Vitalogical "Living Water" foods then other enzyme-rich Protein-Calcium-Phosphorus-Iron Proportions to be used sparingly, and finally going to the anti-enzyme, slaughtered flesh, soups to breads. The cooking of food destroys the enzymes, part of the vitamins and even the protein integrity. On December 26, 1977, the Associated Press published a report affirming that: The National Cancer Institute presented findings by Dr. Abdon that the boiling of food caused Protein Mutations: In addition to their findings earlier that charcoal broiling and baking of food produced hydrocarbons that cause cancer. The Cancer Institute also stated that the combined causes of cancer, such as smoking and alcoholism, produce a multiple cause of cancer, similar to the combined use of more than one kind of pesticide may augment the cause up to 100 times the potency of the original cause.

The cooking of food also destroys the anti-enzymes of decomposition and the reproductive purposefulness of seeds, but due to their chemical composition with affinity to reproductive instincts, the human reproductive excesses are augmented, and toxic decomposition bacteria are nourished, augmenting the auto-intoxication that engenders a whole syndrome of ailments in the most susceptible regions of the body. It matters little whether we cook seed foods and flesh foods or eat them raw as many are advocating today, the toxicity of such soon destroy us.

As to vegetables, legumes or flesh cooked in soups with lifeless water, sensually it simulates food substances suggestive of fresh fruits or vegetables, but the lack of the enzymes of life subtracts from human health with deficiencies in living cellular integrity. Human education teaching the perversion of our original natural appetites has alienated people into believing that raw living food is harmful, and that lifeless cooked and prepared foods that do not decompose readily, are good for mortal beings that require enzyme-motivated action to be alive. Life is destroyed in vacuum packed containers, as well as rapidly cooked meals. Even the addition of salt to foods destroys enzyme action in them.

As we inferred already above, the enzymes of decomposition found in raw slaughtered flesh, like the reproductive enzymes found in seeds, divide and subtract from human life if they are eaten, and cooked flesh destroys even the decomposition bacteria of already dead lifeless substance, which has nothing to add to our living human flesh, and thus wastes our digestive enzymes internally synthesized, and only irritates the body with poisonous stimulation similar to drugs. The animal flesh hormones are subtly hybridizing human flesh, as it is assumed by facts on food assimilation, lowering humans to animal instincts, and much worse the mad demoniacal behavior that makes men fight wars, participate in all kinds of crime and other psychopathic actions common among men now.

The immature growing enzymes of green corn or peas, the germinated plant enzymes of grain and legume sprouts, and the lacto-bacterial enzymes in milk curds, cheese and sourkraut, are in turn like the digestive enzymes found in fruits and vegetables, that perpetuate the health and life in humans. Between 32 degrees and 104 degrees F. enzymes are very active, but above 160 degrees F. all enzymes are permanently destroyed. Beside properties mentioned above, dried alfalfa (lucerne) meal contains enzymes such as Protease, active in digestion of proteins, Coagulase and Peroxidase, acting on the blood, Amylase & Invertase, converting starches and sugars, and Lipase, splitting fats.

On the Island of Majorca housewives prepare curdled milk by beating the milk, stirring it with split fig branches which causes it to coagulate rapidly. Figs contain a protein-dissolving enzyme called ficin or cradein, similar to the enzymes in papaya and pineapple.

In the study of the supremacy of Vitalogical sources of food, back in 1946 on August 26th, there was a report of Vitarian record-breaker in speed, who needless to say possessed none of the bunchy big muscles of traditional athletes. Bedouin tribesmen hunting gazelles in the Syrian desert caught "gazelle Boy" living with animals who grazed on grass and roots. They said he could run at 50 miles per hour, and out raced the Jeep they used on the hunting trip. Caught and tied to prevent his escape, the boy was sent to a Damascus insane asylum. Such human stupidity, to imprison and commit such supermen into medical experimentation, is to be deplored. This herbivorous deer-footed and dieted boy ran nearly a mile a minute or 3 times as fast as the slightly less than 4 minute mile of Olympic Records. Herb Elliot the famous vegetarian Olympic miler ran the Olympic mile in 3 minutes 35.6 seconds, but our mentioned Gazelle Boy had none of the vegetables, dried fruits, and other concentrated health foods Elliot had. It means the simpler grass and root diet of the gazelles provides superior nutrition than all the laboratory inventions in dietetics. More, men are slaves in food habits.

THE WORD OF JESUS TAUGHT FASTING
ON LIVING WATER FOR LIFE EVERLASTING

A fast is defined by Webster's as (1) Abstinence from food, or from certain kinds of food; (2) Time of fasting. The Synoptic Gospels all say Jesus fasted 40 days. Many of the ancient prophets fasted 40 days. But these informants do not state if they fasted with or without earthy water, fasting being assumed to be without food and not from drinking. However, food composition charts will verify that the most essential ingredient of natural living or "raw" food is water as the substance from which life is derived, or as His Gospel says "living water". Earthy inorganic water has its purpose for bathing the body externally, but Living Water is the internal ingredient of life.

John's Gospel gives the final clarification of the meaning of the Bible's Synoptic Gospels. After John gives testimony about the arrival of the Spirit while he was baptizing on the Jordan, those who follow Jesus are described as being John, James, Peter, Andrew, Phillip and Nathanael, men who presumably saw Jesus walking on the shore and heard his teaching as they listened to his witness. John styled his Word of Jesus similar to when God walked in the Garden of Eden looking for Adam and Eve, who had been beguiled by a talking serpent.

Immediately, in chapter 2, John preaches his Esoteric Allegory about the Wedding of Cana, which qualifies in fact as a place in Galilee, but by "Wedding", among Essenes this means the disavowal or forsaking of marriage, since "Cana" means to negate or forsake. The miracle of changing water into wine, is used to introduce his "Living Water" theme since his kind of water is freshly pressed cider or juice from the wine press, this being the best "new" wine, which in Aramaic alternatives also means "fresh" wine which is the juice. This is why John says that the water Jesus gives in the parable or allegory about the woman at the well in Samaria in chapter 4, is "living water" that "springs up into Life Everlasting" which in Aramaic means Salvation. The baptism of Salvation thru Jesus is referred to as the "Lord's Supper" in which again he repeats: "I say unto you, I shall not drink henceforth from this fruit of the vine until the day when I shall drink it fresh with you in the Kingdom of the Father."

Now, in the translations of the earliest manuscripts, in the Didache (The Teaching of the Twelve Apostles), it specifies that the earliest version of Jesus's teaching meant in John's words, "Amen, amen, I say unto thee, Unless a man be born again of living water and the Holy Spirit he cannot enter the Kingdom of God. What is born of the flesh is flesh; and that which is born of Spirit, is spirit." This shows that John and his followers who witnessed the Spirit descend upon those baptized in the name of Jesus Christ were living on Living Water, freshly pressed juice from a wine press. Thus, the fact that Jesus fasted 40 days means that at Cana they lived 40 days on grape juice, which is the life-blood for the manifestation of Jesus, or upon whom his Spirit descends. Thus, in Apocalypse 14 John speaks of the Blood of the Lamb flowing from the wine press which obviously Jesus claims his blood is grape juice (fruit of the vine), and since lamb in Aramaic can also mean the "Prophesied" or Foretold One, this is why one's garments or body must be washed or baptized in the grape-blood of the Foretold Messiah.

As John emphasizes, such living water fasts can be realized with access to cider or wine presses, or other methods of extracting fruit and vegetable juices. Many are familiar with sugar cane mills, or similar ones extracting juice form sorghum or corn stalks, beside the tapping of trees for maple, palm or other sap. In our book "Modern Live Juice Therapy" (1962) we show how hundreds or thousands of people have been healed while fasting taking nothing but carrot, grape, or other fruit and vegetable juices. Dr. Shelton's Health School fasted people using distilled water, just as others used earth water, but our findings have corroborated that fasting on living water develops less suffering and crises beside healing what was often risky to undertake when fasting on inorganic dead water. The inorganic dead water depends entirely on the body needing to synthesize its own enzymes for hygienic health-restoration works, while the Living Water fasting provides the life functional enzymes that enable healing with Life. The weakened or unhealthy body often finds the extra-burden of synthesizing enzymes over-burdensome, while Living Water supports and rests these synthesizing functions, providing water with enzymes for cellular cleansing hygiene, mineral deficiency restoration and general health reparation.

This modern live juice therapy has been promoted by Doctors N. Walker, Kirschner, Gerson, Lust, Szekeley, Brandt, and many others. Such fruit or vegetable juices, having their own digestive enzymes are thus immediately assimilable by the blood, that is in 15 or 20 minutes, resting the digestive and metabolic processes of the human body. In turn, fasting with distilled water which is cooked water, has been shown to also burden the body with Leucocytosis, producing an unbalance requiring great numbers of white corpuscles as a defensive action. Yet fasting with earthy water from springs, streams, wells, etc. introduces inorganic caustic substances like limestone, iron rust, salt, etc. that stiffen the body with deposits giving old age arthritis, and other chronic ailments. No matter how one looks at the Gospel's teaching, the baptism or washing with grape-blood of the Foretold Christ, is the essential foundation for knowing the

Realm of the Presence of God, the Salvation from the weaknesses of the flesh, and Life Everlasting.

The outstanding thing to be gained from fasting 40 days taking only earthy inorganic water is formidable personal will power. When your writer did his 40 day fast on dead water at Lake Quilotoa in 1948 on the last 5 days he was barely conscious without energy enough to think. The secret as to why the great prophets fasted 40 days is revealed in Matthew 17:19 which clearly states: "If you have the faith of a mustard seed, you will say to this mountain, Remove from hence, hither, and it shall remove and nothing shall be impossible to you." Thus, fasting is the very key to the Kingdom of God, in that it makes one a participant of God-Power, Omnipotence of Almighty God!

The psychological factor involves the gaining of power of complete do-minion of the self, or what spiritually may be viewed as overcoming self will with the Divine Will. This was the weakness of Dr. Shelton's Health School, in that people only fasted for personal gain in health. Too often, without the Gospel's objective in mind, they fell back into their old habits unable to achieve the necessary will power. Among the early Hygienists who based their beliefs on the Bible it probably was much more spiri-tually oriented. Fasting has been in professional use in America since 1822, when Isaac Jennings, M.D. used it to treat patients in what he called Orthopathy.

Your writer did not realize his clear understanding of the power of Living water until after his tinctured water fasts. This was due to all information on fasting being based on dead inorganic water. In fact, living on juicy fruits, or even on fruits and raw vegetable salads, it becomes difficult or painful to swallow such inorganic things. To be able to drink water at all it becomes necessary to add some fruit juice to give it an objective, and to eat dead cooked food it requires eating raw salad with it. These pecu-liarities thus fashioned my use of fruit juice to tincture the spring water used in the 1952-1953 fast of 7 months 7 days, and the distilled water used in the 1953-1954 fast of 6 months 17 days. The first tinctured water fast resulted in swelling of the legs due to salt, limestone, iron oxide and other minerals in the spring water that accumulated in deposits faster than the kidneys could eliminate them. The tinctured water fast using over a gallon of water distilled for 99.94% purity eliminated the leg swelling and gave great elasticity and agility to the whole body. However, in the end, it was naturally absurd and ridiculous, to tincture water with minute quan-tities of dietetic tomato juice or immature sour orange juice to be able to swallow a gallon of dead inorganic liquid that nature refused otherwise. Conforming with Nature, the instinct only desired Living Water.

Yet, there were benefits gained even with the tinctured water using spring water, in that in 4 and a half months, the improved metabolism allowed the putting on of weight up to 212 pounds with the greatest strength your writer ever achieved working, lifting and carrying boxes of apples. Starting the second tincture water fast, after 105 days the body had autolyzed the excess fat reserve, with apparently no loss of muscular tissue, and as said with outstanding muscular agility. Such fasts rest the digestive organs from hours of work required normally, yet one is not so weak that bed rest is required, so he can attend to chores sawing fire-wood, do some gardening or typing as your author worked on mostly beside mimeographing his journal and books.

The tinctured water was made with 5 parts distilled water, to one part tomato juice which was 95% pure, so the tinctured water was 99% pure, or about the same mineral content as pure spring or well water. The homogenized solution was warmed on the stove, avoiding boiling, and after drinking in 15 to 20 minutes it was evacuated in a bowel movement of warm liquid that had cleansed the whole digestive tract. Taking this warm internal bath especially on winter days gave the illusion of having eaten 3 times a day and minimized the appetite for food. Yet, at the end of the second tinctured water fast, the body had autolyzed even the muscular tissue to the point that the fingers clasping around upper arm could touch solidly. Obviously, the ideal place to break the fast eating fruit, would have been at about 105 days, before the muscular tissue was autolyzed, having lost the excess fat like the hibernating bears. But even such unnatural procedures, using distilled water, tomato juice in cans, the illusive warm body purges 3 times a day, etc. could be dispensed with if one simply ate juicy fruits and succulent vegetables, or took their juices without excesses. Only the carnivorous beasts and domestic cats and dogs who partake of what humans eat, find that they must fast, the herbivorous and frugivorous seemingly regulating their appetites with resting, or their environment doing it for them. Dr. Shelton continually warned people not to go on long fasts without supervision, which often was judicious, yet the prophets of old removed themselves from people who could interfere, especially family relations, and with God's help did what was needed for them. Eating the fruit-salad diet or living on freshly made juices avoids the appearance of invalidism, and one's neighbors will seek advise as to how they can remain youthful with pleasant roundness of features without hanging, adipose or misplaced flesh, never knowing illness and living generations after one's own contemporaries have passed on. As Jesus said, "Nothing will be impossible for you!" The greatest pitfall among healthmen is the desire for the spectacular, stunting, when really the greatest benefit for health is moderation, taking only what the body needs and avoiding all excesses.

THE SECRET OF VILCABAMBA CENTENARIAN'S LONGEVITY HIDDEN PERHAPS IN ENZYME FACTORS OF THEIR DIET

Morton writing "In The Steps of the Master" described the Temple at Jerusalem: "Thousands of beasts and birds atoned for the sins of humanity at the altar of the Lord. Blood flowed in a never ending stream, and the smell of the Temple was the stench of burning fat... It gave no spiritual direction. It was merely a sacred shambles. Isaiah sounded its death knell centuries before Christ: "For what purpose is this multitude of your sacrifices to Me, saith the Lord? I am full, I desire not holocausts of rams and fat of fatlings and blood of calves and lambs and buck goats." The description of the Temple of Jerusalem parallels the Temple of Vilcabamba when I arrived in 1962. On Sunday, as a Carmelite Tertiary at the time, I was obliged to receive Holy communion. Approaching the church at the right side was a butcher's market in front of the gate to the priest's quarters, displaying the anatomy of swine for sale especially on Sundays and holidays. The Sermon given by the old priest was often centered around my accusations of the backward nature of the local religion, and the elderly clergymen even promoted flesh-eating as good theology. Yet, their faith had degraded worse than at the time of Christ, for not only clean beasts but pigs, the abomination of Jews and Moslems, beside strong drink was the only religious indulgence used to celebrate the holiday obliging Christians to congregate. So disheartening were these practices, that I soon left the Roman Catholic Church to return to the primitive Essene worship of God in private as a hermit, finally abandoning such a sacrilegious "Sacred Valley of Longevity", ironically the title I had promoted Vilcabamba with for 18 years.

The fact that Jose David Toledo, my first neighbor, had a birth certificate due to the baptismal records in this mentioned church, proving him to be born February 12th 1859, was supposed to prove also the longevity of the other centenarians who were his school-mates. Yet, when he died in 1971 at 112 years, the newspapers and tourist propaganda stated he had died at 140 years. Add 1859 to 140 years and you have 1999, when he is supposed to have passed away, which future date we might prognosticate is a time for repentance and confessing such frauds to start the Third Millennium with Righteousness Restored. Every afternoon, after hoeing his patch of yuca, he would rest on his porch smoking his home-grown tobacco, a vice that could hardly give any record longevity beyond 112 years he was certified to be. Actually the oldest centenarian of Vilcabamba, may have gained his long life due to the lacto-bacteria elaborated dairy products, similar to those of Russia, Bulgaria, etc. Manuel Ramon, who lived at least 126 years if not more, was a cowherd when a young boy for a convent of Catholic nuns who had a dairy near where I lived near Vilcabamba.

For over 33 years while living at Vilcabamba and a region 20 miles south we have depended on milk for curds from cows that graze on the mountain-side there, which is above the flatter agricultural lands that are at times contaminated by agro-chemicals. Thus, fresh cheese seems to have been the protein staple before hog raising was introduced with auto roads, so that roast pork became the chief food sold in shop fronts. Cheese, curds and curdled milk products from cows fed grains, sawdust, cardboard and manure and other absurd cattle foods now reported in use in the U.S.A., are sure to give an unhealthy product. Cheese as we have illustrated is a high enzyme food. Another enzyme factor predominate at Vilcabamba, found usually in their centenarians gardens, and with which Manuel Ramon for many years supplied us with, is the creamy mountain papaya called "Babaco". Papayas contain papain, an enzyme that digests albuminoid substances, preventing a great deal of bad effects that cooked yuca (mandioc), beans and corn would give without its use. Papain is another enzyme which digests foreign growths on contact, destroying intestinal worms, warts and even is used in the treatment of cancer. Thus, it is the pepsin and papain that account for the people being able to eat so much roast pork and other heavy proteins today. Another ugly factor that confronted your writer when he arrived in 1962 were the scavengers of human offal, namely swine that freely wandered in the street. Human offal contains enzymes that the body secretes to digest cooked food, and in turn, these people were scavengers of equal parasitical nature that existed upon the hogs they fed with their bodily wastes. Thus, among the various peculiarities found in Vilcabamba was the eating of part of their swine raw, uncooked. At the apartment where I first stayed, every week a hog was slain in the street below, and the parts provided for whoever ate there. Early in the morning the people usually went down to the river to fetch a tin pail of water for their kitchen, and to wash parts of the recently killed pig, beside eating raw pork hide as they merrily gossiped about town happenings. However, the raw pork fat of this "tasty and delicious" pig skin contains the enzyme lipase, which digests fats, and thus shows why Vilcabamba was called "An isle of Immunity for Cardio-vascular Ailments" before I began publishing data on the centenarians.

Again, returning to papayas, they also contain carpaine, another enzyme which digests fats. The lipase in raw pork fat may account for the digestion of the raw food, but the roast pork, plantains fried in pig fat served to tourists, and other so-called delicacies lacking fat splitting enzymes, probably depended on Papaya's Carpaine enzyme for relief. This was effective when Dr. Eugene Payne discovered the lack of cardiovascular ailments among the inhabitants. This fat-tolerance factor really dates back to the time of Ponce de Leon searching for the Fountain of Youth, who discovered Florida, but along with these ambitions it was revealed that natives could ingest such great quantities of fat-ladened flesh because they consumed lots of papayas also.

Seeking the answer to why people in the Vilcabamba region no longer reach centenarian ages, and why already in youth the young people's teeth were rotting in their gums, I found they had a carbohydrate tolerance problem. However, among my workers I noticed there was a youth with perfect teeth without one cavity. Inquiring into his case history I found he came from a nearby valley which as yet then had no access by auto roads, and thus no gasoline engine powered sugar-cane mills. When asked as to what they did in their spare time, he replied that they chewed sugar cane. Other authors have also noticed that people who chewed sugar cane, rather than consume cooked sugar products had fine shiny white teeth. Sugar cane chewed raw abounds in juice rich in enzymes such as amylase, catalase, ereptase, invertase, maltase, oxidase, peroxidase, peptase, saccharase and tyrosinase.

Thus, in their boyhood, these world famed centenarians of Vilcabamba, were in a similar isolation without wagon or auto-roads to Loja, rarely traveling to the city on horseback, and certainly without gasoline powered sugar-cane mills. Your writer also spent considerable time in similar inaccessable regions to auto travel, where animals were used to power sugar-cane mills, and the raw sugar was hauled out on mules. Today, the workers have little time to stand around chewing sugar cane, the rapid grinding of the canes by gasoline motor, making it imperative to rapidly haul in and cut cane fast as one can to earn extra wages. I noticed some fellows never ate lunch, sucking chunks of raw brown sugar all day, while others consumed sugar syrup when they entered the mill shed, and white bread and pastry, formerly unknown to the centenarians in their boyhood, along with white rice, were the everyday staples. Dr. Howell shows the cause of ailments like caries is accompanied by an increase of the size of the pancreas, liver, etc. and the shrinking of brain size, and among these people there were numerous mentally affected or intellectually backward individuals who avoided any schooling beyond 6 years, and spent most all they earned getting drunk or on non-essential novelties, radios, television, etc.

Among the centenarians, we cannot say there was no alcoholism, but this vice seemed to be tolerated by them. Yet, even here the enzyme factor played its part, in that what they drank was a corn-beer called "Chicha" popular in every region of Ecuador. It is made by sprouting corn giving the enzyme amylase which converts starch into sugar, to which fruits were added to give distinct flavors. A similar drink was elaborated by the long lived inhabitants of the Amazon, who had their women chew yuca (mandioc) roots raw so as to convert the raw starch with the salivary amylase. The lack of phosphorus mainly in the soil of the Vilcabamba valley we have elsewhere spoken about, since it adds years to life, altho lacking brain building needs, just as yuca is an easier food crop to grow there than corn requiring more phosphorus. St. John's bread, carob, is of high calcium to phosphorus ratio.

A BRIEF HISTORY OF ENZYME
NUTRITION AND DR. HOWELL'S FINDINGS

The history of enzymes as described by Dr. Edward Howell in his book "Enzyme Nutrition" began with the misadventure of being based on the error that enzymes work by their mere presence, without being used up in the process, which was based on the work of O'Sullivan and Tompson on invertase in 1890. This was contrary to the definition given by Roberts in Lumlian Lectures of 1880, that the living body imparts a definite amount of vital force to enzymes, and that this force acts upon a substrate until it is exhausted, which D"Sullivan and Tompson ignored. "Enzymes represent the life element which is biologically recognized, and can be measured in terms of enzyme activity. Our easiest measurement is a lack, for various chemical reactions fail to occur without enzymes: a radiated or a cooked potato will fail to sprout. Thought of for years a catalyst, enzymes are much more than these inert substances. Catalysts work by chemical action only, while enzymes function by both biological and chemical action. Catalysts do not contain the `life element' which is measured as a kind of radiation which enzymes emit"

Then Dr. Howell shows that its radiations cannot be measured by ordinary devices, but are known as Mitogenic Rays of Gurwitsch, Kirlian Electro-Magnetic Photography, Rothen's Enzyme Action at a Distance and Visual micro-observation of Working enzymes. Enzymes contain proteins and some contain vitamins which can be synthesized by chemists. But the life principle or activity factor has never been synthesized. The carrier of this factor of enzyme activity are proteins. That these enzymes are not exhaustible, as assumed by others, is the argument that Dr. Howell elaborates upon in his book. Dr. Edward Howell, born in 1897, received his medical license in Illinois, spent six years on the professional staff of Lindlahr Sanitarium, a renown nature cure hospital, after which he continued work in his own practice of treatment of chronic ailments using nutritional and physical therapies. He retired in 1970 going to Florida to continue his investigation into enzymes of which he is America's pioneer and foremost biochemist and nutritional researcher. Each one of us is given a limited supply of body enzyme energy at birth, which means the faster one uses it up, the shorter one's life. In fact by using living food, fruits and vegetables with the vital force in the fullest supply, we use up very little of the body's enzymes, enabling optimum long life, which cooked foods and those with enzyme-inhibitors rapidly waste away bringing on disease and old age. There was something seemingly coincidental in the lives of Dr. Edward Howell and Dr. Johnny Lovewisdom. We both became conscious of the enzyme factor of living food early in the 1930's, when even before his vegetarianism, Dr. Lovewisdom took to the old country diet of the Finns, meaning sour milk, dark whole grain bread, vegetables and fruits simply due to his failing health on the conventional diet. In 1935, becoming a vegetarian, and a year later even leaving out eggs and milk products, I went to see a Seattle Naturopath since an eye doctor had prescribed stronger glasses, but the Naturopath prescribed both wheat and rice germ, giving a similar experience as Dr. Howell had experienced in being depleted in strength, revealing the anti-enzyme or enzyme inhibitor factors in reproductive substances when eaten raw.

However, when Dr. Howell announced his findings in his 1944 book, "The Status of Food Enzymes in Digestion and Metabolism", that same year Dr. Lovewisdom read the Holy bible for the first time, which re-vealed to him that the nuts and seeds he had learned to avoid due to their causing of seminal losses, was actually the forbidden food, or "fruit" of the Garden of Eden. In Genesis 1:11,29, it specifically stated that green herbs that yield their seed for propagating their own species, and fruits which likewise yield seed for propagating their own species, were to be man's food and means for building more Paradises of fruits and leafy vegetables. Dr. Howell's findings were of scientific importance, while Dr. Lovewisdom's were of psychosomatic, moral and religious implications in the life-style man should conform with for well being.

However, since Dr. Howell had already begun his experiments on an all uncooked or raw food diet years before Dr. Lovewisdom's physi-cal birth, he certainly earns priority in scientific recognition, while Dr. Lovewisdom's findings were based on bringing spiritual upliftment to mankind, revealing that the precepts on enzymes and enzymes inhibitors or anti-enzymes were the very teaching originating with the beginning when the Elohim or God(s) created man in their own image and likeness. Neither Hygiene nor Enzyme Nutrition have contributed to making man holy or spiritual, but rather promote a challenging problem for those who are unable to conform. This we saw in the Vilcabamba centenarians who gained longevity by eating raw pig fat, cheese, papayas and other high enzyme foods grown on soil rich in pulverized minerals altho low in phosphorus, yet the inhabitants eventually degraded into alcoholism, narcotics, roast pork, and other evils consumed.

As Dr. Howell emphasized, whole nations have lived on raw unpasteur-ized milk, butter, cream and cheese which contain the enzyme lipase, with a high standard of health, longevity and freedom from cardiovascu-lar diseases. Even the Eskimos who live on raw fat and flesh, almost free of carbohydrates have been free of civilized ailments, which set in just as soon as cooked and denatured foods were introduced. One of the commercial schemes to prevent cholesterol formation giving cardiovascular ailments was the substituting of highly refined vegetable oils, which have a long "shelf life" like white sugar, white flour, etc. in supermarkets. Yet, they act only as an anti-cholesterol drug, sending high concentrations of fats to the bowels causing fatty tumors.

A report entitled "Incidence of Cancer in Men on Diet High in Polyunsaturated Fat", Universities and the Veterans Administration in the Los Angeles area collaborated in a clinical trial extending over 8 years to test the efficacy of a diet in which vegetable oils were substituted for saturated fat. The test involved 846 men living in government hospitals. Half of them were kept on a diet with purified, unsaturated fats, while the other half ate a regular diet with ordinary fats, including butter. Those eating unsaturated purified fats had lower blood cholesterol levels and fewer deaths from cardiovascular diseases, 48 versus 70. An unexpected finding after this 8 years of diet was that of the 423 subjects eating the purified fat there were 31 deaths from cancer, while in the 423 eating some animal fat there were only 17 deaths from cancer. In a press conference in 1971, the architects of the program, Drs. M.L. Pearce and S. Dayton, of the University of California issued a warning to go slow both on cholesterol and purified oils.

Concerning the enzyme lipase, the rule of seeds having enzyme inhibitors, in cases, can be ignored in the case of flax seed, wheat, coconut or similar seed foods more tolerable, due to the need of the fat-splitting enzyme lipase, when the seminal loss producing factor becomes less effective with age. Moreover, sesame seed is the only seed that has a higher calcium proportion to the phosphorus (1160 to 616 mg.), altho it has 18.6 grams protein. This resembles Swiss Cheese with 925 mg. calcium to 563 phosphorus and 27.5 grams of protein. Due to such high concentrations of food elements there is a need of multiple quantities of salad vegetables with living water to dilute the excesses with a correct balance in minerals and protein.

Enzyme activity in a seed is at its height when a sprout is approximately one-fourth of an inch long, according to Dr. Howell. From his charts we note that the enzyme inhibitors in seeds such as lettuce is completely neutralized 100% in 24 hours, and in the case of the proteolytic enzyme, Trypsin, it breaks down proteins to amino acids in this time with 60 units of Trypsin. In 72 hours or 3 days, 333 units were broken down, while before sprouting 7.5 units were active, so there was an increase of 52.5 units. In 3 days there was over a six-fold increase or 600%. Animals and humans that are fed soybeans or other seeds, legumes, grains or nuts, thus cause an over-secretion of the pancreas which is lost in feces, wasting the body's enzymes, becoming stunted in growth and sickly. It is only the eating of fruits and vegetables that compensates the regular Hygienists to be in better health than people who live on cooked food that has no enzymes at all. But Vitarians may thus increase their enzyme potential over six-fold by using sprouts. Cooked food soybean eaters really are with a burden similar to flesh eaters, since they neither get the enzyme-inhibitors, nor the enzymes, since cooking destroys all of them, giving a 6 fold burden.

Instead of 120 years, man should live 720 years or even near a millennium like the Pre-Diluvian patriarchs, applying the Paradisian precepts on diet.

The editors of the Scottish Medical Journal stated: "Probably nearly half of our daily production of protein in the body consists of enzymes. Indeed, each of us, as with all living organisms, could be regarded as an orderly integrated succession of enzyme relations." What this means is that our breathing, sleeping, eating, working and even thinking are enzyme dependent, adds Howell. We could not exist without enzymes. Thus, Jesus, Life and Living Water and Food ("bread") all relate to a Living God, since all existence depends on enzymes.

As to who actually coined "enzyme inhibitors" or "anti-enzymes" there are various scientific sources, altho the present writer published his objection to the use of seeds in "Spiritualizing Dietetics,- Vitarianism", in 1954, of which several editions were made in Kaweah California, Delhi India, and Omangod Press in the U.S., so that Dr. Lovewisdom's belief that nuts and other seeds were the forbidden food and original sin in the Garden of Eden in Genesis, was public information, beside the actual experimental evidence he encountered in 1935 and 1944. Thus, it would seem Dr. Howell must have read this book to state in "Enzyme Nutrition", "Tree nuts and other seeds, beans and grains, contain superb proteins and fat intended by nature for the perpetuation of their own species." Thus, this foremost enzyme scientist agrees exactly with this public information contributed by Dr. Lovewisdom as to the Bible's Genesis teaching that seeds should not be eaten in the Creator's precepts given unto men.

In defense of Dr. Howell's affirmations as to who actually coined the terminology, these are his words: "It is obvious that enzyme inhibitors are needed only in the seeds and not in other parts of a plant. But what is required for the well being of seeds poses problems for animals and humans wanting to eat the seeds for food. In 1944, enzyme inhibitors in seeds were discovered independently by E.D. Bowman, Indiana University, and W.E. Ham and R.M. Sandstadt, Nebraska Experimental Station.

Prior to that (approximately 1920 to 1940) scores of chemists referred to "free" and "bound" enzymes in seeds, but did not understand the mechanism of inhibition. It was known that the addition of protein digesting enzymes to seeds would free their enzymes from bondage and increase enzyme activity greatly. Germination did the same."

However, altho I had only a few followers in my fruit diet experiments avoiding seeds in the 1930s and 1940s, by the 1950s and especially by the time Dr. Viktoras Kulvinskas of Omangod Press published my first dietetics, book, thousands were experimenting with our Vitarianism, since I received voluminous mail eulogizing my work and asking for other books I might have written of a similar nature. As a sidelight on the value of enzymes thru-out nature, the system of organic farming speaks highly for the necessity to return to the old-fashioned way of agriculture.

The use of chemical fertilizers, pesticides, weed killers, etc. not only is lacking in enzymes, but moreover is lethal to all life in the soil. Compost of organic materials, mulch, manure of animals and human waste are full of enzymes that give health to living things and especially the fruits and vegetables that we eat.

That Dr. Howell, Dr. Santillo and others promote supplemental enzyme concentrates, thus involving a commercial factor, does not subtract from their proven basic importance, especially when these supplemental enzymes are capable of digesting over a million times their weight in cooked food. This does not solve the problem in reality, since cooked food supplementation is obviously a very around about way of avoiding natural foods and living, and still carries with it many damaging effects on health beside mere food digestion. Only natural living, integrated with the eating of fresh ripe fruits and raw vegetable salads are the true and ecological answers to health.

Now while Dr. Howell did publish "Food Enzymes for Health and Longevity" with Omangod Press a year after "Enzyme Nutrition" was published in 1985, both Viktoras Kulvinskas and Dr. Santillo in their works do not promote pure unpasteurized dairy products, much less cheese as do Dr. Howell and Lovewisdom, but rely on sprouted seeds only rather than both curds and sprouted foods. However, this is due the antecedent troubles Lovewisdom has with hypoglycemia predominate for the 33 years he lived in the tropical highlands below and south of Loja city, where bananas and other sweet fruits excessively prevailed as everyday staples. As already described the high calcium phosphorus and proteins with enzyme concentration of curds and cheese greatly relieved the hypoglycemia, was the easiest and purest solution, and satisfied the body's craving in making large bowls of salad palatable. Of course, sprouts are recommended as an alternative, altho in severe cases of the intestinal lacto-bacterial flora being incapacitated by toxic agro-chemicals or drugs it still proved a life saver as it was for your writer. Also, one's choice may depend on whether it is easiest to get seeds to sprout from organic sources, or milk for curds or cheese that is free form antibiotics beside the agro-chemicals in the cow's fodder.

Sprouts are high in amylase which converts starches into sugars, but had plenty of amylase, maltase and sucrase, so the amylase enzyme has nothing to do with the hypoglycemia problem. But bananas, all seeds, beans, grains and their sprouts have higher proportions of phosphorus to the calcium, except sesame seeds and most milk products especially cheddar and Swiss cheese. Milk contains the most enzymes of any food, especially in the lacto-bacterial products mentioned, except sugar cane which is another hypoglycemia provoker, of which Howell lists Amylase, catalase, dehydrogenase, galactase, lactase, oleinase, peroxidase and phosphatase. People with hypoglycemia become afflicted with osteoporosis and other mineral deficiencies, or lack lipase if they use salad oils and the other enzymes not mentioned above that digest fats and proteins. In 1945 when the author lived a year in Quito, and fruits in the market were not treated with agro-chemicals, he experienced exceptional health eating a great variety of fruits including avocados, tomatoes, mangos, apples, papayas, pineapple, bananas, plums, oranges, to which he added cauliflower. His cheeks were plump, just as I have seen other fruitarians especially women acquire, but after the coming of agro-chemicals and the use of drugs, the many fruitarians visiting us at Vilcabamba were thin, nerve-wrecked and weak specimens of what in other times had been super-health.

There is a great difference between the weight of people and animals that eat cooked foods without enzymes, and those who eat uncooked fresh natural food, in that cooked food is excessively fattening. Obesity is a common ailment among civilized people in our world. Many people consider the food calory content of bananas, avocados and seeds before sprouting when cooked as equal to the natural uncooked items. Cooked food is fattening, because it over-stimulates the endocrine gland. For instance it would be useless to try to fatten animals with raw potatoes, or put on weight in humans eating them raw, while cooked potatoes can put on excess weight as your writer's experience has proven. However, such excess weight was pathological, not coordinated with the health of individuals. Potatoes cooked produced a heavy sediment in the urine due to the coagulated albumen in what is known as albuminuria. Raw potatoes are delicious to persons who eat numerous raw foods that release the starch blockers in digesting them, so they serve as a vegetable in salads.

In a work by Paul Kouchakoff, M.D. "The Influence of Food Cooking on the Blood Formula of Man" (Institute of Clinical Chemistry, Lausanne, Switzerland, 1930), the eating of cooked food, and even the consuming of cooked water (teas, distilled, etc.) was scientifically proven to augment he white blood cells, known as leukocytes. This condition is described as Leucocytosis, which Webster's describes as "an increase in the number of leukocytes in the blood; it is a normal occurrence in digestion, and during pregnancy but a pathological condition in infections, anemia and certain fevers". Phagocytes are defined as any leukocytes that digest and destroy other cells, microorganisms or other foreign matter in the blood and tissues. Phagocytosis, thus is identical to leucocytosis, coming from "phago" or phage, meaning eating or destroying. Autolysis is the destruction of cells or tissues by substances within them, as after death or in some diseases; this condition thus is what occurs in phagocytosis. Whether this is "normal" in occurrence in digestion as Webster's puts it, thus can be scientifically disputed, since by simply eating natural uncooked and unprocessed food, there was no substantial increase in phagocytes. As already explained this process is carried on with digestive enzymes that "eat" or consume the cooked food or other foreign disease producing substances in the blood and lymph fluid in the body.

Thus, what herein is illustrated is that the destruction of enzymes in natural uncooked food, greatly taxes human or animal organisms by having to resynthesize the needed enzymes in their digestive processes, so that the immunological system is soon debilitated, giving the common childhood ailments, beside the recent appearance of cancer, SIDA, cardiovascular diseases and other pathology in children, beside the increased occurrence among adults and the elderly. This reduces the length of life and the quality of our well being among a universally cooked food eating and ailing race. The large pancreatic gland, is still not large enough to possibly produce all the enzymes found in the muscles, glands and tissues and cells of the body. Nearly half of our daily production of protein consists of enzymes, and 400 grams of body protein is degraded and resynthesized in the body every day. Obviously, food can only provide the least part of these 400 grams, human milk having only 1.2 grams, meaning that lysosomes filled with digestive enzymes which aid in amoeboid-like digestive processes of multicellular organisms are responsible for this. Lysosomes were discovered by the electronic microscope, altho the processes of phagocytosis was visible with ordinary microscopes, showing the engulfing and digestion of food substances or foreign micro-organisms by the blood. This shows that old worn out cells of the body, as well as the dead cooked food, are resynthesized by autolysis. Abstinence from all food allows the autolytic disintegration of pathological tissues such as tumor and other abnormal growth, a process observed by Graham already in the middle of the 19 century, altho it is also observed often with the giving up of cooked foods and natural living in general.

We have already observed how the many enzymes in papayas pre-digest its food elements, beside proteins, fats and other food substances in other foods eaten at the same time. Just as figs (with ficin) were a standby eating fruits in California, pineapples have been my favorite and most health restorative fruit in Ecuador. The digestive enzyme, bromelin, in pineapple relieves the body with function of two body enzyme secretions. The acid digestive secretion in the stomach, pepsin, starts the digestion of protein, but for the need of an alkaline medium the protein food goes on to digest in the small intestines with trypsin, a pancreatic enzyme. In the past, these two enzymes were extracted from animals for therapy of digestive ailments in humans. However, various biochemical investigators found that bromelin had an active range from 3 to 8 in pH, or is able to continue digestion from an acid environment in the stomach to the alkaline media of the small intestines. Thus, bromelin effectively does the work of pepsin and trypsin, with one enzyme. Both Drs. Howell and Santillo have shown plant enzymes to be even more capable than animal extracts, and certainly more natural to the Creator's intended design.

Also pineapple has an ideal balance, high in calcium, 17 mg., to 8 mg. of phosphorus and only .4 grams of protein.

Adele Davis, called the foremost nutritional authority, has insisted that animal liver is basic for having nutritional balance. Excessive in phosphorus, 362 mg. to 10 mg. calcium, it has nearly 20 grams protein. Descriptions often given as to animal liver being alive and shaking with cancer, but desiccated who will know the filth and disease inherent in such a biblically unclean flesh. (However, had Dr. Alexis Carell used a healthy liver as the source he derived his immortality cell tissue instead of a chicken's heart, this might have gained great commercial value as a pseudo "Health Food".) As it was, relying on liver she died of cancer before average non-health-conscious Americans, like the pill-popper J.I. Rodale who depended on such toxic supplements. My criticism is not against much good they did for a healthier world, but as to why they could not break their attachment to flesh food.

Now, that we are on the subject of an immortal elixir, enzyme re-synthesis and living water, we might give a better solution than the recent concentrated supplements. In the papaya tree family is a plant that produces not fruit, but the leaves are used as greens since instead of being bitter like papaya leaves these are agreeable. It is called "Col de Monte", but is neither a cabbage nor related to mountains, but rather a wild jungle growth, altho it survives in arid regions also where it is used for hedge-like live fencing. The more you cut it, the more it grows. Wherever you find it you usually find chayotes, which is a single seeded fruit of a vine that covers trees, and whose fruit can be baked like squash when old and starchy, but young and tender it takes the place of cucumbers in a salad, or is fine as an extender giving living water in juice. So you take col de monte leaves and cut sticks from the chayote and run them thru a juice extractor, and you have the finest "Elixir of Immortality" Milk Shake. Escarole, celery and other greens can be mixed in for a delightful combination. The milky sap of this col de monte digests parasites and tumors, and the papain and pepsin digest protein, the carpaine digests fats, while other enzymes with minerals and vitamins join with living water in the tender chayote to digest carbohydrates to purify the body's cellular composition. America has yet to discover this fountain of eternal life.

For almost a century, free parcels of corn flakes, bran and even laxatives arrived in every mail box thru-out the United States, and billions were spent to advertise all kinds of "junk foods" which had their health virtues removed, and are now believed to be responsible for the poor health of Americans. Now, a new trend is initiated in selling the concentrated wheat germ, minerals, vitamins and other ingredients people were cheated out of having for their health by the 100 billion dollar food industry. However, the missing link to health is in everyone having their own backyard garden and orchard providing an untampered with source of living food and rejuvenating living water. When Yogis and other esoteric students go into a trance such as Samadhi, they are able to bring about a standstill in the life processes of the body: the heart slows down to an imperceptible pace, so does the breathing, and thus does also the grosser aspects of metabolism and mitosis, preventing decay of the body. Even in fasting, cellular division is at a minimum and life processes are nearer to rest at an easy pace. With a diet furnishing living water to cleanse the cells and give living nourishment, the cells of the body are slow in change, like Dr. Alexis Carrel's chicken heart tissue, which he cleansed with distilled water tinctured with vinegar, and was found capable of infinite division and life. But with the acceleration of cellular division consuming more concentrated nucleic acids from the protein of seed foods, liver, flesh food, etc. the body rapidly wastes away with habitual wear and tear for the enjoyment of food and consequent sexual stimulation.

Now, all we have said about enzymes in living food and living water, the autolysis and resynthesis of the cells thru-out the body, and so forth, is what the Apostle and Evangelist John preached nearly two millenniums ago. What could be more specific than: "Unless a man be born again of living water and the Holy Spirit (Breath, Wind) he cannot enter into the kingdom of God." Just as the fruit of the vine or juice he pressed from grapes, and his (St. John's) bread, are described as his blood and flesh, the Spirit of Jesus said thru John: "Unless you eat the flesh of the son of Man, and drink his blood, you shall not have Life in you." That flesh, bread or food in Aramaic, he said was live, sent down from heaven, just as the Heavenly Man made in the image and likeness of God was commanded to eat only succulent herbs and juicy fruits that yield their seed for propagating and growing their own species. "Search the Scriptures, says John, for you think in them to have Life Everlasting, and the same are they that give testimony of me... In the Beginning was the Word..." John's word continually tells you to refer to the first chapter of Genesis to know what and how man should live. Science only invents new words and ways to say the same thing without remembering the Divine Source.

Another aspect in Life Conservation, meaning the preservation of enzymes, comes by eating local foods and living in the "land closest to the sun", Ecuador to be precise at the Andean equatorial regions, the potentially most healthful and spiritually heavenward "Land of Eternal Youth". This your writer was intuitively inspired to make his home, spending his first 8 years around, or within in the latter 4 years, the crater of an extinct volcano, by Lake Quilotoa. The "lake within the peak of a mountain" arrived at by spiritual direction was 12,600 feet above sea level, the top of the crater being at 13,000 feet. The lake being of warm springs origin averaged 60 degrees F. or 16 C. so altho being at an altitude usually having frequent frosts, on the lake shore tomatoes ripened and it was frost free.

In robust health your writer often hiked barefoot on the mountain tops white with frost bare headed, or in winds strong enough to toss a native from a horse. I reiterate these details at present to explain conditions where the body's enzyme supplies are conserved in the cool super altitudes since the life processes are slowed down, just like in the hibernation of animals. There are less heart beats, slower deep breathing and there is the least of aging or wear of the body.

In turn at low altitudes, the temperature is higher, the body perspires faster than sweat evaporates, the heart beats faster and one tires faster working. Like in the Finnish sauna in mid-winter it is warm and relaxing at first, but the circulation soon spreads up and soon the skin eliminates the body's wastes by copious sweating. However, if you spent over an hour with all the heat you can stand in a hot sauna, the body's enzyme supply would become exhausted, and a person may faint. As Howell points out the enzymes start being destroyed at 118 degrees F. So, by providing 46 F. temperature daphnia magna were able to live 108 days, but in the warm 82 F. temperature they only survive 25 days. Of course humans who I have known to live 120 years in the Quindigua lowlands on plantain soup, will not live 4 times as long at super altitudes high in the Andes, except if they lived on juicy fruits or a similar raw foods diet. The 120 year woman was exceptionally frugal, so that at a mile high in the Andes at Vilcabamba, men who lived pleasurable lives with much more bodily abuses, also claimed to often reach 120 years, while their parents were bragged to be very old including a woman of 150 years. However, the reason the inhabitants at the super-altitudes were a small race of no out-standing longevity was because they lived on cooked barley nearly alone, lacking enzymes. The lack of enzymes in food points to the fact that they, like people who live without eating, perhaps got their enzyme sources from the air they breathe, containing bacterial life, altho it greatly limits them, if there is any effect at all.

This conclusion I came to observe due to the fact that people that were known to live without eating (see "Spiritualizing Dietetics,-Vitarianism") only lived the same amount of years, usually less than 70 years, as did the average cooked food eater, even at high altitudes. However, observing the greater longevity of animal life and humans at higher altitudes meaning cooler temperatures, along with the strict diet of fruits and raw vegetable salads, explains why your writer moved from his mile high Shambhala Sanctuary in Loja province to Cuenca in Azuay province at about 8,400 feet altitude. Unable to heal a ruptured disc in his spinal vertebrae in six months, and asphyxia often noted on warm days at the comfortable tropical altitude with a great variety of fruits in production, beside threats on his life at the time, the change involved considerable sacrifice, but once at the higher location, with the change to an almost exclusively vegetable salad diet, brought steady improvement in what had become an intransigent condition.

The bacteria in the air require an alkaline high calcium food like cabbage and milk to develop lacto-bacterial culture that gave longevity to the centenarians in Vilcabamba, Bulgaria, Russia and in the exception of the Hunzas it may have been the uncooked apricots and mineralized soil of the high altitude. But, living without eating still uses up the body's own enzymes.

However, since we mentioned people living without eating average the same length of life as cooked food eaters, means the body's own enzyme supply is used up whether we resynthesize the gaseous elements in the air, or resynthesize the dead cooked food, both of which wear away or age the body's enzyme potential. Thus, let us reiterate the facts on the life of Saint Nicolas Von der Flue, the patron saint of Switzerland, who lived an exemplary life as a family man according to worldly standards, raising five sons and five daughters. When he was 50 years of age he was inspired to take up the life of a hermit. Many people protest when one speaks about the solitary life, excusing themselves due to their responsibility in raising a family, earning a living, but Jesus did not tell us for nothing that we must forsake our home, land, wife, sons, daughters, mother, father and life in this world. Nicolas Von Flue obtained the consent of his darling wife, and leaving his 10 children, the youngest only 6 weeks old, having explained his need for meditation alone, left everything. Thus, he spent 20 years living as a hermit in the Swiss Alps without food, dying on his birthday March 31st, 1487 at 70 years of age. Altho he weekly went to partake of the Eucharist which is a paper thin wafer, this had practically no food value. In the 50 years of his earlier worldly life, the use of Swiss cheese probably prepared a good stability in health, so by then inspired by the Gospel, he gave up everything, even food for religion.

the flesh that carnivores eat. What more, if flesh is cooked or any living food is heated much over 129 degrees F., the enzymes are sterilized or destroyed. What we do by such action is annihilate or waste the enzymes which are limited in the amount of life they contain. By cooking or sterilizing the life in food, the consuming human body is forced to produce the necessary correspondent enzymes to digest and metabolize such dead foods where-in life has been sterilized. From this comes the Genesis of childhood diseases, the epidemics of ailments in human life and the rapid aging and death among humans.

However if men and women return to eating living food, the living bread in the Aramaic interpretation of Jesus, the vital energy of the body no longer is wasted in synthesizing enzymes that are destroyed by cooking and no longer do we have the cause of disease and aging in the measure that we are able to apply this into practice in our lives.

Moreover, even beyond life as effective energy in vital actions, enzymes have intelligence as to how to fashion and make live, transmute the nutritive substances into our flesh and body so as to renew our anatomy continually, from one instant to another and thus revealing this to be Life itself, and not some vitamin or substance that man can imitate by synthesizing a similar chemical.

To illustrate the characteristics of enzymes, I am going to tell you about an experience that happened while I was writing this thesis. We were preparing for a trip to get to know some regions near Cuenca to buy apples or other organic fruits, and so it was necessary to see that there would be no bother as to bowel movements due to my lower extremity paralysis. Dr. Mujahed my companion and attendant in getting my food and other needs, had noticed that the use of cheese from Cayambe which seems to have more enzymes and to be most free from antibiotics and other toxic chemicals because it is made of milk from cows which graze in the highest mountain regions of Ecuador and thus is "hoarded" by the intestines in a constipation that seeks the utmost profit from the use of enzymes that are found in this protoic substance in calorie concentration. Like the ripened cheese such as Swiss and Cheddar of U.S., the Cayambe varieties, (mozzarella etc.) are concentrated enzyme supplements, with greater metabolic harmony for assimilation since their calcium content exceeds the phosphorous content, calcium being the digestive king-pin followed by other mineral concentrations, while fresh cottage and similar curds tend toward lesser to lacking enzyme concentrations of fresh milk, which like unsprouted seeds contain nutritional enzyme inhibitors. The mention of cheese from Cayambe, Chedder or Swiss should be modified to say "without salt" or "low in salt", since this chemical, sodium chloride, is a protoplasmic poison, a dangerous irritant and a cause of cancer and for this reason destroys life in enzymes similar to cooking. The bodies of the mummies in the pyramids in Egypt were preserved with salt for many thousands of years because they contain no life since their enzymes have been used up and prevented from returning as in normal decomposition of dead corpses.

Also he had observed that if bananas are eaten in abundance daily to help in bowel movements, or when there is a tendency toward constipation this maintains regularity. The excess of bananas may produce hypoglycemia especially if vegetables are lacking, there is a tendency to have a drippy nose and also there is mucosity that enables bowel movements without the use of enemas without difficulty in separating the compact and hardened mass. Thus David Mujahed with doctorate in Vitalogical Sciences served me only a small slice of cheese with a dish pan sized bowl of lettuce, cabbage, celery, grated carrot and tomatoes. I did not wish to protest at the moment but the cheese lasted me to only half the salad taking a crumb with each bite of salad.

The other half I had to eat with bananas for calories, altho I had a bowel movement accomplishing our objective. Yet, all that night I suffered from spasms and cramps because I had been tempted to eat an apple beside cabbage in less degree of chemical contamination from pesticides, altho I had eaten of the same cabbage that was slightly toxic but had had no painful spasms. Thus, I discovered that the portion or slice of cheese contained sufficient enzymes to cancel the effects of the pesticides, enabling the use of vegetables that people ordinarily use from markets with no painful effects because they have the ability to synthesize enzymes in their liver and other organs to cancel the effects.

Many people today take massive doses of vitamin C so as to avoid the
need to stop smoking, just as I had abused the abundant use of cheese
to cover up the use of vegetables more or less poisoned with pesticides
inadvertently. Actually, it is not possible to eat apples from the ordinary
markets without being poisoned more or less. David and Patricio also
had indigestion or other similar effects. In my case, being of greater age
and lacking in enzyme potential of the liver, in consequence I had painful
spasms and cramps beside nightmares in which bandits threatened by
life. The next day I recovered tranquility after a meal of certified organic
vegetables without pesticides and cheese in an abundant double portion.
Altho it is not advisable to eat a lot of ripened cheese in the years of one's
youth due to excess of protein, in this age of contamination and poisoning
of almost all food sold in markets world-wide, this is the only medication
effective against the deadly effects of toxic effects of food sold in regular
commerce.

Thus, there is a source of profitable industries for the production of food
without pesticides, herbicides, chemical fertilizers and other factors that
are mining the public health. With popular demand the markets will
begin to help the consumer in place of exploiting them with "foodless
foods" lacking nutritional value, and filled with the "weeds" or causes of
cancer, heart disease and other imbalances that are produced by the way
of life and habits now in fashion in our civilization and the lack of culture in our "scientific" age in relation to the Tree of Good and Evil in our
world.

Another observation at this writing was the surprisingly purifying reaction that the large bowls of cauliflower (favorite), along with green leaves
finely chopped, lettuce, tomatoes of certified organic sources, beside
carrot, beet with tree tomato juice at lunch, had replacing the cells of the
body formed from deficient diet and environment and removing a large
quantity of uric acid and other wastes coloring the urine, in a visible
process of rejuvenation. With paralysis of lower extremities, the feet were
cold for lack of assimilation so with a hot water bottle warming the feet,
the great amount of waste deposited in the feet loosened and with ability
to metabolize the vegetables a rejuvenating cleansing thus ensued.

Now what do our investigations have to do with yoga, self-realization and the Breath of Life which is the foundation upon which Oriental Science rests. The Science oriented in Breathing claims that to breathe is to live, but physiologically the respiration oxidizes, and thus integrates the carbohydrates and other substances in the process of metabolizing food and synthesizing cells, tissues, organs and the body with the soul, which depends upon enzymes with their intelligence and vital action in life itself.

The famous Yogi's of the twentieth century such as Paramahansa Yogananda, Swami Sivananda of Rishikesh and many more, in the observations of learned people today in the field of nutrition and physical fitness, are heavily burdened with adipose flesh, regardless as to the tradition among Yogis that corpulence is a special gift in the spiritual life of masters.

So, just like taking vitamins to cancel the effects of smoking and using cheese for enzymes to cancel the effects of toxic agro-chemicals, these famous yogis were utilizing hyper-ventilation to oxidize the sterile cooked diet of rice, chapatis, legumes and similar foods. That they were storing "prana" or vital energy was dependent upon enzymes which are to be found in natural food without cooking as known from the beginning of man, but eliminating life from their food, the yogis need to recur to breathing exercises to store vital energy so as to synthesize enzymes by physiological processes in the digestive organs. Consequently, the Natural Vitalogical Sciences are with greater orientation as to life and the initial Godly Creation and its millennial consummation, than the Oriental Sciences themselves in this orientation. Since man was told just what was the prohibited fruit which were the seeds of fruits and vegetables which in turn are enzyme inhibitors or anti-enzymes, and what man should eat to keep his intimate communication with God, he has had the Breath of Life, in body and soul, ever since his Creation in likeness and image of God. Therefore for a natural and divine Breath of Life, without artificiality or artifice in Pranayama, we should be fed on wholesome enzymes of the Spiritualizing Dietetics of Vitalogic Continence as in the original Paradise of Divine Design. There is no need to rectify the Respiration, or the effect, but rather we should obey the first commandment or precept given unto man, that we are to eat juicy fruits and succulent vegetables, and thus in the Creative Communion we shall have Natural Pranayama, the true Breath of Harmony with the Paradisian Life.

In the Paradisian Lifestyle by its communion with God the Creator the Elohim the Word and Son of God and the Heavenly Realm of God in Divine Design, man returns again to enjoy his original Tropho-Euphoria, the Paradisian Blessings of living in the Presence of God.

THE SCIENCE OF SPIRITUALIZING DIETETICS FOR THE ATTAINMENT OF VITALOGICAL CONTINENCE

In our South American perspective reviewing some vegetarian health magazines from the United States, the predominant interest of the follow-ers of Natural Hygiene stood out especially in "Alive and Well", which we support in other aspects except in it's dedication to having babies and pregnancy of their mothers. In our point of view and criteria, the over-population and environmental pollution due to concentration of excessive human population, and the lack of plant life and vegetation to provide for the breath of life and human nutrition, indicates the urgent need for the health and quality of life on our planet, in a lifestyle exemplifying the limitation of population and promoting the appreciation of chastity and continence as the remedial means against more and more pregnan-cies and lives centered in the production of more infants to suffer in the misery of human over-conglomeration and environmental pollution. The value in the quality of life exceeds the quantity of sentient beings strug-gling for survival with a lack of provisions for living. This is why the Dietetic Science with a Spiritualizing perspective in place of the common proclivity of animals in reproducing an abundant offspring, promotes the absence of such carnal attachments and bestial instincts in continence just as has been idealized by the religious celibates among Catholics, Bud-dhists, Yogis and others. The solution has also been given in the Sacred Scriptures. When man and his wife ate the seed of trees instead of the true tree fruit, the ingested substance augmented the human seed, proving that sexual shame and the obligation of bearing children is the result of eating the seeds of fruit and herbs in place of the real fruit and vegetables. The reproductive and food enzymes are opposites in function, or inhibi-tors of their opponents. The food that was prescribed by the creator is for a healthy long life of the consumers, but the reproductive food substances divide and subtract to multiply their number who become competitors in using up environmental resources reducing more and more the quality of their food. It is for this reason that for half a century your author has pro-scribed seeds of all kinds, including nuts, which the natural hygienists, recommend, and consequently causes their great concern about pregnan-cy and their babies, and their belittling the spiritual life. Moreover, the "Alive and Well" magazine articles include some against the use of milk and it's products, which in reality condemns the modern dairy industry

146

has fallen far below the quality standards of former beside modern health concerned producers of cheese and other milk derivatives equal in quality to other certified organic foods.

THE VITALOGICAL ENZYME
PATH TO NIRVANIC EMANCIPATION

As an avid anthropologist, and the author of "MYSTICAL ANTHRO-
POLOGY CONSTITUTED AS A FUNDAMENTAL VITALOGICAL
SCIENCE", I feel the necessity now of reconstructing a synthesis of the
prudent wisdom of accounting for the intimate oneness of the origins, in
the teachings and the objectives of the Essene Christ, Jesus, and the Ma-
ha-Bodhic Buddha, Siddhartha Gautama. Both Philo of Alexandria and
Flavius Josephus, as the foremost Essene historians contemporary to the
original Christian or Essene Apostles, described the Essenes as originating
in northeast India, thus indicating their inception in Buddha's homeland,
and of their basic monastic philosophy. The Christian Apostolic Fathers,
Hippolytus, Epiphanius, Eusebius, and others frankly admitted that the
Christian New Testament and tradition was identical to the Essenes, or
complained that the Primitive Christians adhered to the Eastern Buddhist
so-called heresies, as we have elaborated in the "Buddhist Essene Gospel of Jesus." We also show that the Nazarene or Nazarite (identical in
Aramaic) Vows of the Christian Essenes identify with those of the Early
Buddhists.

With this historic preview, I have sought to identify my mission in rein-
carnating Ananda, the beloved cousin of the Buddha, Siddhartha, and
John, the Apostle Beloved of Christ, whom the other Apostles among the
Twelve followed, and whom St. Thomas Aquinas described as the very
Hypostasis of the Word and Son of God, Jesus. Now, in the symbolic
33 years that I lived in Loja Province of Ecuador, as we described in the
biographical synopsis in the preceding international publications about
the "Saint of the Andes", we have told about our International University
of the Natural Vitalogical Sciences, and the incorporation of the "Pristine
Order of Paradisian Perfection" along with the "Heavenly Ecclesia of
the Living God in Aeonian Revivification", in which we thus legalized
the teaching of the Vitalogical Sciences in Ecuador. So now our task is to
illustrate how our Paradisian Order will relate our past to the present and
adapt to our new home in San Joaquin suburb of Cuenca.

Bethany House of Shambhala Sanctuary we named to illustrate the Maha
Maitreyana Mandala, or the new World Spiritual Center, transferred
from Tibet and the Himalayas to the Equatorial Andes, prophesied by
the ancient Buddhist Scriptures after the decease of the 13th Dalai Lama.
Even the details of the Buddha's reincarnation coming from the region of
Seattle, as illustrated with Bernardo Betolucci's film "The Little Buddha"
for all to see are a confirming manifestation. Bethany, Aramaic for Fig
Gardens, on the Jordan identified the desert climate of the Baptist and
Apostle John's hermitage, was transferred to the climate and the flora

of our former Bethany House of the Shambhala Sanctuary, since the east and west boundaries were described living Bodhi Trees, so that sun's illumining orbits were described therein by these old Bodhi fig trees. They we surmise were brought from India as cuttings from the original at Bodhi Gaya by Buddhist missionaries sent by King Asoka before the Christian era, just as papayas, bananas, sweet potatoes and other food plants are believed brought to America long before Columbus and our Christian era even. The Buddhist art with lotus, swastika, and dragon designs, beside the long eared, red top notch statues are also identifying characteristics. The Buddha realized Nirvana under the Bodhi fig tree, after he decided to partake of a catalytic enzyme food, perfumed curds brought by a dairymaid, who either used fig sticks to curdle the milk, or the Buddha elaborated his meal by adding the wild fig which parrots like and humans in need sometimes eat, containing ficin which digests the curds in the food-enzyme stomach.

As to John's food on the Jordan, it was carob meal combined with bananas, since Musa Paradisiac and Musa Sapiense, the main varieties were so named because in Aramaic the fig and banana are the same word. Being too warm, altho a desert, real figs do not fruit well in the Jordan trench near the Dead Sea, so one must go like John and his Apostles to the source of the Jordan in the snows of Mt. Hermon, the true Mt. of Transfiguration since it is the only "great high mountain" to locate where true figs grow. The Book of Adam and Eve states "Seth and his most righteous and holy tribe that ever lived" lived exclusively on fruits such as found on their Holy Mountain, Hermon, foothills of which produce fine apricots, peaches and figs. Thus, this now identifies our new "Santuario Monte Hermon" in the garden suburb of Cuenca where we also shall grow figs, peaches, apricots, apples, mt. papayas, loquats, avocados, cherimoyas and tomatoes, just as possible in the San Joaquin Valley of California where we lived many years ago in the foothills of the Sequoia region, enjoying the tradition of Seth, who was also called a Son of God, like his tribe and the followers of John.

Now, we have another parallel as told in the Life of Buddha by Ashvaghosha Bodhisattva, in which Devadatta seeing the remarkable excellence of the Buddha, conceived in his heart a jealous hatred and sought to kill him in various attempts such as rolling a stone down a mountain at him, and releasing a drunken elephant to trample him. We have described in earlier "Chats" about the fellow who repeatedly made various assaults on the author's life, the last threat being May 15th 1996 when we escaped from Shambhala Sanctuary to start our exodus to Cuenca. So due to Karmic consequences, as the Gospel teaches, he who lives by the sword shall die by the sword, and planting bad figs we shall harvest bad figs, my would be killer met his own violent death. As to the "land of milk and honey" of the Old Testament, the Soncino Chumash version of the To-rah explains this as the meaning of Canaan region of Palestine being the land of fig trees and date palms, since figs have a milky enzyme used to curdle milk, while the palms are tapped for honey-like syrup called honey, beside giving nectarous date fruits, while John's "camel hair and hide" garments are a bad translation of the rope-fiber obtained from the palms written and appearing the same as Camel's raiment. The Nazarite vow would not permit John to touch corpses of camels of which hair and hide are a part, Josephus confirming John's abhorrence to being near a corpse. We also describe "The Unknown Life of Jesus Christ" by Nicolas Notovich copied from an ancient contemporary history of Jesus's hidden years from 13 to 29 years of age, which include his study at a Buddhist monastery where it was recorded.

Thus we have elaborated the intimate Buddhist-Christian connection which illustrates why your writer thus presents Vitalogical Enzymes as the ingredient catalyzing Nirvanic and Heavenly Salvation; which influ-enced the Enlightenment of Siddhartha Gautama to become the Buddha at Bodhi Gaya, and the Enlightenment of John, the Essene Hypostasis of the Word and Son of God, Jesus Christ on the Jordan, transfigured lu-minously on Mt. Hermon, home of the Holy Tribe of Seth. For Salvation in today's polluted environment no longer needs the antiquated Yoga system of storing Prana by breathing exercises, wherein due to ignorance, the human bloodstream was polluted with a diet lacking enzymes ingest-ing cooked denatured foods that must be oxidized by respiration, now requires the correction of methods with the Vitalogical Sciences using Enzyme foods high in calcium as the king-pin in mineral proportions found in Chlorophyll of plants which is a generator of the needed oxygen to directly clean the bloodstream upon assimilation. These Survival Tech-niques for the Third Millennium Paradisian New Age we now outline:

THE VITALOGICAL ENZYME
AND CHLOROPHYLL CONNECTION

Proteins with genetic purpose in seed matter were not designed by their nature to be eaten as food, altho they may contain potential life and intelligence as reproductive enzymes. Herein, the enzyme inhibitors or anti-enzymes theory may be misinterpreted, since it may be taken to infer that seeds lack enzymes, when in reality they abound with them. What is meant, is that seeds lack nutritional enzymes of immediate utility to humans when ingested, since their enzymes are the reproductive enzymes of the germ and the stored starchy carbohydrates, fats and proteins that become available, unlocked or uninhibited when the seed is sprouted, releasing the enzymatic potency in sprouts. It is like the egg of barnyard fowls, in that the white genetic material which is transformed into the chicken, etc. is nourished by the yoke when hatched, but inhibited or inassimilable to humans. This is why raw eggs are used to provoke vomit, until some humans learn to ingest them just as other toxic substances are accustomed by perverted habit.

Every living thing on earth survives, perpetuated in Life Everlasting, ever-changing, forever reborn anew and ever passing away, to reappear in regenerated Continuity. The Buddha Siddhartha, like Krishnamurti in our time, sought to put an end to Continuity, but perhaps did not realize that the Karmic purposefulness of trees, plants, animals as well as humans when interfered with, or intercepted, continues bonds in this eternal Continuity, whether we call it perpetuating Karma of Reincarnation. Eating rice, bread, etc. made from grains, legumes, nuts, eggs, or genetic cell substance of animal flesh, whether used cooked or raw, interfere with the Almighty's purposefulness in Creation and Nature, and is bound to intercept consequences in health physically, beside psychologically and spiritually. The Creator was the Word, the Wisdom, by which all that was created was made, and altho an abstract God, yet manifests illusively in the good and evil consequences of our actions.

Thus, Vitalogical Hygiene has a Spiritual Teaching that illustrates our ultra-modernity today, yet is down to earth in being based scientifically in the food enzyme concept, but applied by practice, without the need of marketing enzyme supplements to better the lives of our followers. Whether we kill enzymes by cooking them in our food, or we use the foods raw in their natural state, in the case of seminal substances in all seeds, beside eggs and slaughtered flesh foods, we are partaking of food enzyme inhibition, or anti-enzymes, since neither dead inert cooked enzymes, nor contrary purpose enzymes of reproduction were ever intended for nutritional purposes. Ultimately the fruitarian gospel is the Karma free life of Liberation, the Emancipation into Nirvana, breaking with Continuity in suffering derived from errors in actions whose consequences are not foreseen, and thus overcoming selfishness for Selfless Enlightenment. No matter what humans indulge in, they live in bondage of some habit or "addiction" that eventually destroys them. A slave to our contemporary civilization, eating flesh, consuming inert cooked food and other stimulants of sensual appetites, very few have ever succeeded in overcoming this world built upon suffering.

Our New Testament preaches it, as did the Sutras of the Buddha. Today the majority of Christians and Buddhists, no longer would ever want to give up the attachment to their forbidden, Karma-adhering everyday foods they endearingly ingest for sensual pleasure. It provokingly humiliates our human dignity, our over-estimated intelligence, to someday contemplate and realize what fools we are in ignoring common facts. This is the Omniscient purposefulness in designing human beings in such habitual adherence to sensual pleasure. How ridiculous may our race remain in filling their bodies with lifeless pasty pap that obviously adheres to and clogs one's insides, various gluey substances to obstruct the blood circulation, if not bury unsepultured corpses of our fellow sentient beings? What shame: even observable among the corpulent adiposity of religious monks and nuns, Catholics, Buddhists, Yogis or whatever, what they are, speaks so loud of their erroneous life that the world is incapable of hearing or adhering to their message.

We are about to enter a New Millennium, and for the sake of the Christ, the Buddha or whomever we esteem as ideal exemplars, it is time to put an end to this perpetual blasphemy of God and good common sense. How can a person be a Temple of the Holy Spirit, when the fat of fatlings, pork, beef or sweet griddlecakes and the like are the host worshipping Yahweh disguised as Lord God? 'Tis time to throw out the butchers, fish mongers, bakers and other sea cooks of perverted savory dishes from the Temple of the Holy Spirit. If a man truly remembers his Maker, he should at least do so when he partakes of what he shall become. Feeding on swine and foamy sponge we call bread, what else shall we become?

Recently in Ano Cero magazine from Spain there appeared a review of the film of "The Road to Wellville" about two of the great Hygiene institutions of America. The famous surgeon, Dr. John Harvey Kellogg is in it, claimed to have invented the breakfast cereals marketed by his brother, peanut butter and the electric blanket. Battlecreek Sanitarium, the largest in the world as we have described, was actually founded in the late 1800's by the Seventh Day Adventists, a vegetarian religious group. They put John Harvey Kellogg in charge of it in 1876; jealousy arose between them due to the personal fame of the illustrious physician. The Adventist leader Ellen White had a vision of a flaming sword over the famous sanitarium, and consequently the wooden building was burned in 1902 to fulfill the prophetic vision. The well produced film with actors is about a young couple who are confronted with what is called a "fascist" health regimen which lends itself to an entertaining comedy. Since it relates to the pioneers of the Hygienic Medical foundations in America, of which the Loma Linda medical school still graduates physician, and the Adventists are a prominent religious church, the review of it intrigued us. Could anything be more fantastic than the 20th century monopoly and dictatorial policies of pharmaceutical-surgical medicine and physicians? In turn the practice of Hygiene engenders confidence and sure-footedness unequalled by other systems provided it is really genuinely vitalistic and naturistic.

Our theme of the Enzyme Path to Nirvana, much like our sudden thrust removing us from our Peaceful and Fruitful Shambhala Sanctuary to face the reality of the polluted and forsaken civilization prominent in city life, inspired us with the only answer as to how to cope with irony of a "smoggy Breath of Life". This sarcastic emphasis as to the Breath of Life is basically to those living in air polluted environs, that, while the practice of Yoga breathing exercises was acceptable or recommendable in lonely hermitages in the pure air of the Andean or the Himalayan super-altitudes, it becomes threatenly the "Breath of Death" in the polluted cities. Yet, in those lonely pure environs, the almost illiterate people drinking and threatening the lives of others for funds to buy liquor, chose not to practice Hygiene or study the wisdom thereof. In turn, those receptive to the wisdom of hygiene are bound economically by multi-circumstantial air, water, food and psychologically polluted environments. We are not financial wizards, only knowing how to live.

The city's "Breath of Death" multiplies the manyfold effects of Chlorination and other pollutants in the water used to wash our bodies and our foods, just as it is not easy to find organic vegetables for salad and biological fruits. During the day one suffers a quivering or pulsation under the right eyelid, blackouts in vision or headaches, and probably many more irritations difficult to account for if one is eating cooked and chemically contaminated foods of the ordinary diet. After the traffic subsides at night, one greatly appreciates the green lawns, trees and plants with chlorophyll that give forth oxygen of the parks, residential housing areas with small garden, etc.

Considering that the lack of oxygen and the carbon monoxide pollutants are one's basic problem, one must breath the least of the polluted air by conscious mental control first. The late Dr. Teofilo de la Torre, before settling in Costa Rica when I met him in 1938, kept his San Francisco California apartment window closed to avoid air pollutants. Its seemed imbecile for which reason I avoided the city for better air, but on the country farms, due to the spraying of lethal insecticides, I was likewise poisoned even worse, altho my Sequoia Retreat removed me from pollution and communication with the world I was seeking to help. Dr. de la Torre's Edenia magazine was well printed and reached more readers, while my few hundred sporadic subscribers to the mimeographed Eternal Youth

Life, found it hard to live up to my teaching living in polluted cities often. Organic food sources were also scarce.

However, today even in Ecuador, in North America and Europe, the basic organic fruits and vegetables are available in supermarkets, or sellers at organic farms, this helps alleviate the organic food problem as well as the air pollution crisis. Since it is the CHLOROPHYLL within green leafy vegetation that provides the OXYGEN and purifies the air, why keep them at a distance from our body and blood circulation, which the air may thus pollute. Rather we should place these green leafy sources within the body, and in touch with our blood stream for direct assimilation without toxic pollutants. This is the logic in the eating of large salads of green vegetables, since the greens are put thus directly into our nourishing life fluids with the oxygen factories, and life forces of enzymes that enliven and move our being.

Now the Yogis call the life force in the air Prana, but today a vicious cycle is generated in that the Prana-impregnated oxygen has been crowded out or vitiated with deadly pollutants. Yoga is an obsolete science, fully inept for survival, and deadly to city practitioners. Moreover, rather than congesting our bloodstream with coagulating albuminoids, cooked starchy paste or pap, cholesterol-forming fats, etc. let us initiate a new western system of Yoga by breathing thru the enzyme-stomach and digestive assimilation to nourish our blood circulation and enzymatic regeneration of all the cells of our body. With chlorophyll oxygen factories in contact the blood purifies.

Breathing polluted air poisons the red blood cells, just as cooked food and water dissipate the life energy of both the red and white cells so that the red cell mortality increases due to the monoxide gas and lack of organic iron of chlorophyll for the hemoglobin and the white corpuscles or phagocytes increase to remove the foreign blood pollutants dissipating the bodies enzymatic potential. Uncooked living food provides the enzymes and the ventilation or digestive respiration, plus integral cellular respiration that is needed to survive in cities, until one is economically situated to be able to obtain a small parcel of land to grow one's own Paradise and unpolluted sustenance. In the view of oxygen economy: Allowing plant chlorophyll oxygen factories to disperse their valuable gas in the "four winds" it is no wonder we lose a great deal of it beside let it be vitiated with carbon dioxide, carbon monoxide, and the like, while bringing the oxygen generators within the confines of the enzyme stomach none of the precious oxygen is dispersed haphazardly allowing the enzyme intelligence factor to seek from it what formerly it depended on the lungs to furnish, especially in the case of the cooked food and flesh eaters.

Observing these factors, Vitarians should be capable of gaining many more Olympic championships, as illustrated about vegetarians in "Those Strong, Powerful and Extraordinary Vegetarians".

To finish the process, rather than use the forced expansion and contraction of the lungs in Yoga Pranayama exercises, we use the observational conscious method of contemplating respiration taught by the Buddha. Without forcing the breath, mentally we observe the inflow and the outflow, and thus contemplate the implication of absorbing the wide cosmic unbound energy and substance within, and expelling the carbon dioxide and waste products of our metabolism for the fertilization of the plant world that values it, in exchange for the oxygen and chlorophyll minerals beside food enzymes. Thus allowing the enzyme's intelligence to direct the subconscious, or rather super-conscious proclivity contemplatively, we avoid the excess of air pollutants and take in all the oxygen possible from the air as well as the food of our diet.

To profit most from the chlorophyll ingested, chlorinated water must be avoided, since chlorine is another protoplasmic poison with an affinity to vitiate chlorophyll assimilation, beside being known to destroy the intestinal flora, making it necessary to take in much more lacto-bacterial foods. Ordinary chlorinated city water requires a charcoal filter to neutralize the chlorine, but until one can have it installed, one can collect tap water in an open vessel from which it will slowly evaporate into the gaseous form, or boiling also liberates the chlorine.

Another caution that one needs to observe is in reading newspapers and magazines recently printed, since printer's ink today contain instant dryers and pesticides that poison one's blood by mere contact or touch, not to speak of blackened fingers one notes from news hot off the press. By wearing rubber gloves one avoids direct contact with the ink, and it is advisable to wash one's hands before eating, ignoring the advise of Jesus in Matthew 15:20. Even worse in Ecuador there has been a habit of wrapping food in a newspaper unaware of the poisonous ink.

Dr. Ann Wigmore and Dr. Viktoras Kulvinskas have already published the benefits of chlorophyll in wheat grass especially thru-out the U.S.A. Having pots of wheat grass between the watcher and the television tube diverts the injurious X-rays according to Dr. Wigmore, and we might add that being in a room with grass grown from sprouted wheat grain and other plants purifies the air and provides oxygen. If one feels symptoms of air, water or food pollutants, rather than succumb to depression and desperation, chew a little wheat grass and plant more trays of chlorophyll carriers for your survival.

INSTEAD OF WARS OVER RELIGION,
WHY NOT A CONCORDANT BIBLE OF ALL FAITHS

At the time of writing this certain prophets are quoting the prophecies of
Nostradamus and matching the conflict in Bosnia and southern Europe
between Moslems and Christians, as the beginning or the seed of World
War III. As we have promoted in Spiritualizing Dietetics we would seek
to bring the world together by avoiding all but the sublime writings of
the Old Testament, and making an international concordance of a Cosmic Universal Bible, using Christian, Buddhist and Brahminical Holy
Scriptures, and supplemental Scriptures from Islamic, Taoist and other
religions. Much more harmonious and concordant love among humans
might be found without the past obsession for the instructions of Yahweh
the Hebrew tribal God, and contemplating teachings of the Koran, etc. as
we shall briefly illustrate, concordant to our Gospel translations.

As Thomas Carlyle points out "Islam means in its way Denial of Self,
Annihilation of Self. This is yet the highest Wisdom that Heaven has
revealed to our Earth." Thus in the Koran we find concordance using
Christian teachings, and Carlyle calls it a kind of Christianity.

"And Zacharias took care of the child; whenever Zacharius went into
the chamber to her, he found provisions with her; and he said O Mary,
whence hadst thou this? she answered, this is from God: for God provi-
deth for whom he pleaseth without measure. Then Zacharias called on his
Lord, and said, Lord, give me from thee a good offspring, for thou art the
hearer of prayer. And the angels called to him, while he stood praying in
the chamber, saying, Verily God promiseth thee a son named John, who
shall bear witness to the Word which cometh from God, an honorable
person, chaste, and one of the righteous prophets."

"Then the angels said, O Mary, verily God sendeth thee good tidings,
that thou shall bear the Word, proceeding from himself, his name shall
be Christ Jesus the son of Mary, honorable in this world and in the world
to come, and one of those who approach the presence of God.... Mohammed is no more than an apostle, the other apostles have already deceased
before him... For that they have not believed on Jesus, and have spoken
against Mary a grievous calumny; and have said, Verily we have slain
Christ Jesus the son of Mary, the apostle of God; yet they slew him not
neither crucified him, but he was represented by one in his likeness...."

There were many Gnostic Gospels about Jesus, of which four were only
chosen by the 4th century organized Church, and thus they used some
and abused others called Gnostic Gospels, so that Mohammad's version is

much like Paul's, both claiming to be apostles of God. We should not be disputing and fighting wars over concordant versions of Holy Scriptures, since parallels can be found thru-out all the world's religions. Beside some of what Mohammed calls "secret history" we quoted above about Mary and how John bore witness of Jesus who spoke his Gospel from the mouth of John, we now quote from the Koran, a similar incident to John's Gospel (11 and 12) as to Jesus loving Mary, Martha and Lazarus (meaning the Swathed man, Simon) of Bethany. Actually, according to Gnostic sources there was a third sister Ruth, who was not mentioned in the New Testament, disputing over who loved Jesus in serving food or listening to him at the Fig Gardens of Bethany.

"When Paradise shall be brought near, every soul will know what it hath produced. Surely among delights shall they dwell who have feared God; rejoicing what the Lord hath given them... Seated on bridal couches they will gaze around." The wide-eyed damsels which Mohammed speaks about, whether on bridal couches or the chaste relationship of Jesus to women is one in Spirit, since Mohammed acknowledges this as a virtue in John who was the oracle of Jesus's Word. The Buddha also had women as friends donating fruit groves and served them curds in their begging bowls, to supplement the fruit.

"Bowing down at Bodhisattva's feet (Nanda) reverently offered him perfumed curdled milk, begging him of his condescension to accept it. Bodhisattva taking it, partook of it at once, whilst she received, even then, the fruits of her religious act. Having eaten it, all his members refreshed, he became capable of receiving the Bodhi; his body and limbs glistening with renewed strength." Buddha's experience with Mara the devil is like Jesus's struggle with Satan's temptations.

Now, the author's own experience is nearly identical to the Buddhas, due to his 30 years abstinence from the use of dairy products. As an experiment, I partook of clabbered milk and the next morning after a long illness due to malaria, I was able to get up, climb a hill singing the tune "The Last Rose of Summer" which I improvised into "Tis the last Lotus of Shushumna left blooming alone," as I suddenly I entered Samadhi in which all nature shone brightly like a techni-color cinema. This is further elaborated in my autobiography and other books.

However, the curdled milk of which the Buddha Siddhartha and I partook, gave such overwhelming strength physically, mentally and spiritually due to the concentration of enzymatic life energy, and the protective lacto-bacteria that consume the harmful bacteria. I also noted how pineapple and papaya, limes and naranjilla likewise helped overcome the malaria fever, without damage to kidneys, inner ear, etc. that quinine produces. Cooked foods increased the phagocytes of the blood causing an ulcer on my cheek to fester with a mess of dead phagocytes being expelled in a losing battle. However, after climbing a tree with thorns insensitive, and other feats in the trance witnessed by friends I lived with, I was frightened and refused to partake more of the clabber, altho if I had prudently continued just eating raw food, I would have been healed already in those jungles. Man is heir to treasures beyond belief, yet squandering the life force of enzymes, the minerals in chlorophyll rich green leaves, and the Living Water of nature he exists in poverty. +